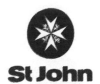

St John

FIRST AID

D0439596

First Edition

REFERENCE GUIDE

St. John Ambulance

SAVING LIVES
at work, home and play

www.sja.ca

First Edition — 2011
2nd Printing – Nov. 2011
3rd Printing – Mar. 2012

Library and Archives Canada Cataloguing in Publication

First Aid:Reference Guide, formerly published as
First on the scene : the complete guide to first aid and CPR. — 4th ed.

Includes index.

ISBN 1-894070-54-2

1. First aid in illness and injury. 2. CPR (First aid). I. St. John Ambulance

II. Title: First aid : first on the scene.

RC86.8.F59 2006 616.02'52 C2006-901819-7

St. John Ambulance

1900 City Park Drive, Suite 400

Ottawa, Ontario, K1K 1A3

Canada   Printed in Canada

613-236-7461   Stock No. 6504-11

www.sja.ca

These resources were developed in accordance with the International Liaison Committee on Resuscitation (ILCOR) Consensus on Science. ILCOR members include the American Heart Association (AHA), the European Resuscitation Council (ERC), the Heart and Stroke Foundation of Canada (HSFC), the Australian and New Zealand Committee on Resuscitation, the Resuscitation Councils of Southern Africa (RCSA), and the Inter American Heart Foundation (IAHF).

St. John Ambulance

St. John Ambulance is a worldwide non-profit, non-denominational, multicultural, charitable organization committed to the service of others. St. John Ambulance is one of two foundations of the *Most Venerable Order of the Hospital of St. John of Jerusalem.* The other foundation is the St. John Ophthalmic Hospital in Jerusalem, which specializes in the research and treatment of eye diseases, and which St. John Ambulance in Canada supports.

In Canada, St. John Ambulance is a national, voluntary agency founded over 125 years ago. Our mission is to enable Canadians to improve their health, safety and quality of life by providing training and community service. The work of St. John Ambulance in Canada is carried out by two groups:

◆ —uniformed volunteers who provide first aid coverage at public events, deliver community health promotion services, and provide emergency response for disaster relief. Therapy dog members provide pet visitations at seniors homes, long term care facilities, children's hospitals etc.

◆ —medical professionals, program development specialists, and instructors who provide first aid and health promotion courses to Canadians

About us

◆ We were established in Canada in 1883

◆ We serve over 300 communities across Canada

◆ We have over 25,000 volunteers who provide two million volunteer hours annually

◆ We train more than 550,000 Canadians in first aid and CPR each year

◆ We are a Canadian Order headed by the Governor General as Prior, and the Queen as Sovereign Head

◆ We support humanitarian relief efforts across Canada and around the world

Contacting St. John Ambulance

St. John Ambulance welcomes your comments and suggestions for this manual. Please write, fax or
e-mail us at the following address:

Client Services
St. John Ambulance National Headquarters
1900 City Park Drive, Suite 400
Ottawa, Ontario, K1J 1A3
Canada

fax: (613) 236-2425
e-mail: clientservices@nhq.sja.ca

Visit the St. John Ambulance
World Wide Web site on the Internet at:

http://www.sja.ca

Emergency Phone Numbers

Police _____

Fire _____

Ambulance _____

Poison Control _____

Emergency Contact

    Name _____

    Phone _____

Home Phone _____

Street Address _____

_____

CONTENTS

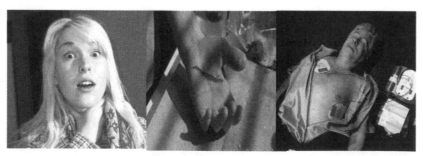

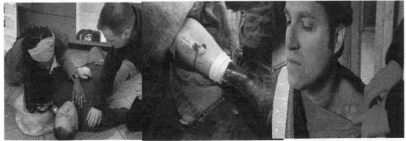

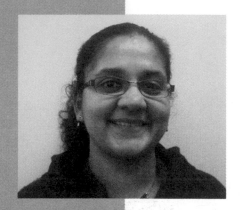

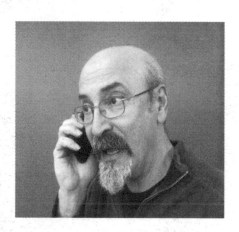

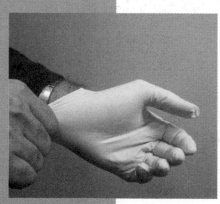

CHAPTER 1

INTRODUCTION TO FIRST AID

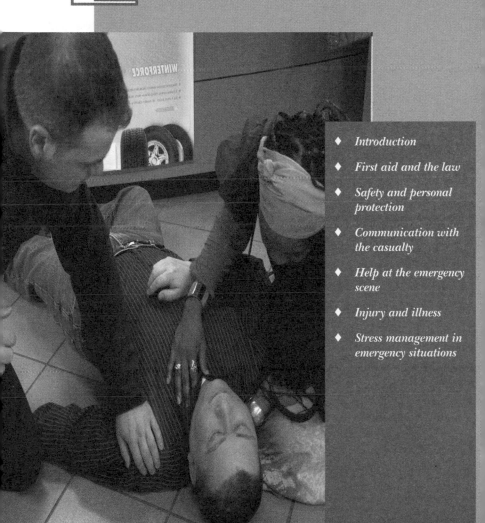

- Introduction
- First aid and the law
- Safety and personal protection
- Communication with the casualty
- Help at the emergency scene
- Injury and illness
- Stress management in emergency situations

1

This guide covers a wide range of information that will help you respond appropriately in a first aid or medical emergency. The introductory chapter contains background information, definitions and other material related to giving first aid. Chapter 2 explains Emergency Scene Management including issues that relate to assessment of the casualty. This chapter also includes topics that are important to understand in the first critical moments at the emergency scene. Chapters 3 to 7 cover a variety of specific first aid topics. Chapter 8 deals with issues of particular interest to health care providers—responders with a specific duty to respond within the health care system. The final chapter includes quick reference charts, a brief overview of human anatomy as well as a glossary and index.

What is first aid?

First aid is emergency help given to an injured or suddenly ill person using readily available materials. It can be simple, like removing a sliver from a child's finger and putting on a bandage, or it can be complicated, like giving care to many casualties in a motor vehicle collision.

No matter what the situation, the objectives of first aid are the same:

◆ preserve life

◆ prevent the illness or injury from becoming worse

◆ promote recovery

First aid is made up of both knowledge and skills. The knowledge is found in this book and can be learned by studying it. First aid skills are different. The best way to learn first aid skills is to take a recognized course from a qualified instructor. In an emergency where there are injuries, your ability to act calmly, assess the situation and give appropriate first aid will depend on your first aid skills. At St. John Ambulance, we strongly recommend you take a first aid course to better prepare yourself to respond in the event of an emergency. Knowing what to do could save a life.

Who is a first aider?

Anyone can be a first aider. Often the first aider at an emergency scene is someone who was just passing by and wanted to help. A parent or guardian can be a first aider to her child, a firefighter can be a first aider to an injured person, and an employee can be trained as a first aider for her place of work. A first aider is simply someone who takes charge of an emergency scene and gives first aid.

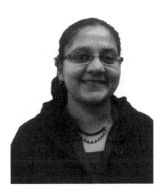

First aiders don't *diagnose* or *treat* injuries and illnesses (except, perhaps, when they are very minor)—this is what medical doctors do. A first aider *suspects* injuries and illnesses and gives *first aid.*

What can a first aider do?

A first aider gives first aid, but can also do much more. In an emergency, where there is confusion and fear, the actions of a calm and effective first aider reassures everyone, making the experience less traumatic.

Besides giving first aid, it is important to:

- ◆ protect the casualty's belongings

- ◆ keep unnecessary people away

- ◆ reassure family or friends of the casualty

- ◆ clean up the emergency scene and work to correct any unsafe conditions that may have caused the injuries in the first place

1

A casualty's age in first aid and CPR

In first aid and cardiopulmonary resuscitation (CPR):

◆ an **infant** casualty is under one year old

◆ a **child** casualty is from age one to age eight

◆ an **adult** casualty is over eight years of age

These ages are guidelines only; the casualty's size must also be considered.

Note that St. John Ambulance is not giving legal advice here. This guide is not intended to replace advice given by a lawyer.

First aid and the law

Can a first aider be sued for giving first aid? Fear of being sued is one of the main reasons people don't help when help is needed most. As a first aider, there are two "legal" situations in which you might give first aid. First, you may give first aid as part of your job—for instance, as a lifeguard or first aid attendant. Second, you might simply be a passer-by who sees an emergency situation and wishes to help an injured or ill person.

Giving first aid as part of your job

When giving first aid is part of your job, you have a legal duty to respond to an emergency situation at your workplace. You have a duty to use reasonable skill and care based on your level of training. This might include more than first aid—you may be trained in rescue, driving an emergency vehicle, etc. If you are a designated first aider at work, make sure your certification is always up-to-date. If you can, take a level of training higher than the minimum—you will be a more confident and effective first aider.

Giving first aid as a passer-by

In Canada (except Quebec) and most of the United States, you do not have a legal duty to help a person in need—if you do not help an injured person, you are not at fault. But our governments recognize the **Good Samaritan Principles** and want to encourage people to help others. These principles protect you if you choose to help someone in need. Once you begin to give assistance, you are obligated to use reasonable skill and care based on your level of training.

Giving first aid in Quebec

The Quebec Charter of Human Rights and Freedoms declares that any person whose life is in danger has the right to be helped. This means that you are required to help a person whose life is at risk, provided you do not put your own life, or anyone else's, in danger.

Principles of the Good Samaritan

You are a Good Samaritan if you help a person when you have no legal duty to do so. As a Good Samaritan, you give your help without being paid, and you give it in good faith (meaning you're helping because you care about the person and not for some other reason). Whenever you help a person in an emergency situation, you should abide by the following principles:

◆ you identify yourself as a first aider and get permission to help the injured or ill person before you touch her—this is called **consent**

◆ you use **reasonable skill and care** in accordance with the level of knowledge and skill that you have

◆ you are not **negligent** in what you do

◆ you do not **abandon** the person

Consent. The law says everyone has the right not to be touched by others. As a first aider, you must respect this right. Always identify yourself to a casualty and ask for permission to help before touching her. When you arrive at an emergency scene, identify yourself as a first aider to

1

the casualty. If you are a police officer, nurse, first aider, etc., say so. Ask if you can help. If the casualty says, "yes," you have consent to go ahead and help. If the casualty doesn't answer you, or doesn't object to your help, you have what is called **implied consent,** and you can go ahead and help. There are some special situations:

◆ If the casualty is unresponsive and relatives are present, ask for consent from the casualty's spouse or another member of the casualty's immediate family.

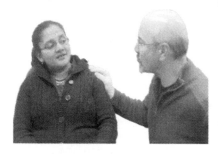

Although it might not seem to make sense that you would identify yourself to an unresponsive person and ask for consent to help her, this is what you must do. Always ask for consent before touching a casualty. If there is no response, you have implied consent to carry on and give first aid.

◆ If the casualty is an infant or a young child, you must get consent from the child's parent or guardian. If there is no parent or guardian at the scene, the law assumes the casualty would give consent if she could, so you have implied consent to help.

A person has the right to refuse your offer of help and not give you consent. In this case, do not force first aid on a conscious casualty. Even if you do not have consent to touch the person and give first aid, there may be other actions you can take, like controlling the scene and calling for medical help.

Reasonable skill and care.   As a Good Samaritan, when you give first aid you are expected to use reasonable skill and care according to your level of knowledge and skills. When in question, care that is given will be measured against what a reasonable person with the same level of knowledge and skill would do. Give first aid with caution so that you don't aggravate or worsen an injury. Make sure you only try to do what you know you can do, and that all your actions help the casualty in some way.

Negligence.   When you give first aid, use common sense and make sure your actions are in the casualty's best interest. Negligence presumes the first aider knowingly acted against the casualty's interest. For example a first aider who intentionally risks the life of the casualty may not be protected. Simply put, give the care that you would like to receive if you were in the casualty's position.

Abandonment.   Never abandon a casualty in your care. Once the casualty accepts your offer of help, do not leave her. Stay with her until:

◆ you hand her over to medical help

◆ you hand her over to another first aider

◆ she no longer wants your help—this is usually because the problem is no longer an emergency and further care is not needed

In summary, there is no reason not to help a person in need. By following the guidelines above, you will minimize the risk of being held negligent for your actions.

Safety and personal protection

1

The number one rule in giving first aid is, "ensure safety." Emergency scenes can be dangerous and you have to make sure your actions don't put you or anyone else in danger. Take the time to look for hazards and assess the risks of any actions you take. You don't want to become a casualty too!

There are three basic types of risks to be aware of:

- **the energy source that caused the original injury—** is the mechanism that caused the original injury still active and could anyone be injured by it? For example, where an injury has been caused by machinery, is the machinery still running?

- **the hazards from secondary or external factors—**are other conditions present that could be a hazard? For example, at the scene of a car crash, could you, the casualty or bystanders be at risk of injuries caused by passing vehicles?

- **the hazards of the rescue or first aid procedures—**is there risk of someone being injured by the rescue and first aid actions? For example, if the casualty is much larger than you are, and you have to move that person, can you do so without injuring yourself?

Preventing infection

A first aider and casualty are in very close contact with each other when first aid is given. This close contact means that an infection could pass from one person to the other. This risk of infection is a safety hazard a first aider always has to be aware of.

There is more risk of serious infection when blood and other bodily fluids are involved, as the viruses that cause AIDS (acquired immunodeficiency syndrome), hepatitis B and other illnesses may be present. Always use **personal protective equipment** (PPE) where available to minimize the risk of transmission.

Steps a first aider can take to reduce the risk of transmission include: hand washing, wearing gloves, minimizing mouth-to-mouth contact during cardiopulmonary resuscitation (CPR) or artificial respiration (AR) and the careful handling of sharp objects.

Gloves   Disposable gloves prevent direct hand contact between the first aider and the casualty. Wear gloves when you might touch blood, bodily fluids, tissue or anything that has come in contact with one of these. Put on your gloves as you approach an emergency scene. Non-latex gloves should be used because some people are allergic to 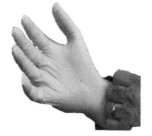 latex. Keep your gloves in a place you can get to easily, where they are not exposed to very hot or very cold temperatures. It's a good idea to keep a few pairs of gloves in your first aid kit. See page 18 for the correct method of removing and disposing of used gloves.

Hand washing   Hand contact is one of the main ways infections are transferred from one person to another. Wash your hands with soap and running water immediately after any contact with a casualty. It is also a good idea to wash your hands often when you are around people who are sick with a cold, the flu, etc.

1

How to remove gloves

Once gloves have been used, they are contaminated and are a possible source of infection. Take them off without touching their outer surface following the steps below.

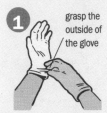

1 grasp the outside of the glove

Grasp the cuff of one glove.

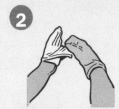

2

Pull the cuff towards the fingers, turning the glove inside out.

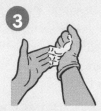

3

As the glove comes off, hold it in the palm of your other hand.

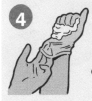

4 do not touch the outside of the glove

Slide your fingers under the cuff of the other glove.

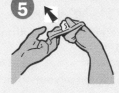

5

Pull the cuff towards the fingers over the first glove.

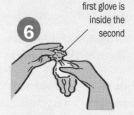

6 first glove is inside the second

Tie a knot in the top of the outer glove and dispose of properly—see below.

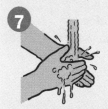

7

Wash hands with soap and running water as soon as possible.

Torn gloves

If you tear your gloves while giving first aid, take them off right away. Wash your hands if possible, and put on a new pair of gloves.

Proper disposal

Seal the used gloves in a plastic bag and put them in your household garbage.

Check with a health professional or your first aid instructor for specific regulations in your area.

1

Minimizing mouth-to-mouth contact   There is always a risk that an infection could be passed from one person to another during mouth to mouth contact (either when giving cardiopulmonary resuscitation (CPR) or artificial respiration (AR)). Use a special face mask or shield designed to prevent disease transmission. Many brands and types of masks are available. Choose a disposable mask or one with a disposable one-way valve. Keep it in an accessible place where you can get it quickly. Follow the directions that come with the mask to use it properly.

Sharp objects   If a sharp object touches infected blood and then pricks or cuts you, you could become infected. Although first aiders do not routinely use sharp objects like scalpels and needles, there may be a need to use a knife or perhaps clean up broken glass that has been in contact with blood. In these cases, wear gloves and handle sharp objects with extreme care. A torn or punctured glove increases the risk of infection.

Safety measures are key to protecting both the first aider and the casualty. Although it may seem like you are wasting precious time by pulling on gloves or getting your face mask ready, this is not the case. Safety is the most important concern while giving first aid. Protect yourself and ensure the safety of everyone at the scene.

Cleaning up after an emergency   Protect yourself while you are cleaning up by wearing disposable gloves. Goggles may also be required to protect yourself from contamination due to splashing. When treatment is finished, all disposable objects must be discarded in an airtight bag. All sharp or cutting objects must be handled with care and stored in closed rigid containers. Reusable supplies and equipment must be cleaned and disinfected according to the manufacturer's instructions. Work surfaces and sites where

1

first aid has been given must be cleaned with hot soapy water or antiseptic solution. A solution of bleach and water in proportions of 1 to 10 may also be used. Blood-stained clothing can be washed with hot soapy water for a minimum of 25 minutes or dry-cleaned.

Anyone who has been exposed to possible contaminants should take a hot shower with soap and rinse thoroughly. Anyone who has been exposed to contaminants from a needlestick or sharps injury should seek medical attention.

Safety in a violent situation

Violent situations are not uncommon. If there are injuries, your skills as a first aider can be valuable. In any emergency scene be on the lookout for violence. If there is violence, or the potential for violence, **be careful**. Your first priority is to protect your own safety—don't put yourself at risk. You are more valuable as a first aider than as a casualty!

Whenever injuries occur through violence, a crime has been committed. If you think a crime has been committed, call police to the scene. While waiting for the police, do the following:

◆ protect your safety, and the safety of others if you can

◆ give first aid for any injuries, being sensitive to the casualty's emotional state (see psychological first aid for assault, page 332).

◆ keep onlookers away as much as possible—do what you can to protect the privacy of any casualties

◆ leave everything at the scene as is—you may disturb evidence that could help police in their investigation

As a first aider, you may have additional information the police will find helpful. Remain at the scene until the police say you can leave. Answer all questions the police ask of you.

Child abuse

When giving first aid to a child with injuries, be on the alert for signs of child abuse. Child abuse is any form of physical harm, emotional deprivation, neglect or sexual maltreatment which can result in injury or psychological damage to a child. To detect possible child abuse, look for signs such as:

◆ suspicious injuries

◆ unusually shaped bruises or burns

◆ apparent fear of the parent or caregiver

If you suspect child abuse, do not accuse anyone. Insist that the child receive medical help for any injuries; this will permit a full medical assessment. If you don't think the child will be taken to a doctor, call an ambulance and the police to the scene—this will ensure a doctor sees the child.

If medical care for the child is refused and calling for an ambulance and/or the police is impossible, call a child welfare agency (often the Children's Aid Society) and report your suspicions. When you make such a call, you don't have to give your name if you don't want to.

Communication with the casualty

When you arrive on scene you may encounter conscious and/or unconscious casualties as well as bystanders. Your communication skills and style will play a critical role as you take charge of a scene. At an emergency scene people can be frightened, anxious and even angry. The first aider can help control the situation by using effective communication skills. Demonstrate competence, confidence and compassion at all times.

1

Always introduce yourself and ask for the casualty's name. If it is an older person they may wish to be addressed as Mr. or Mrs. and not by their first name. Whatever they choose to be called, continue to use the casualty's name through all conversations.

If a casualty refuses treatment, or insists she is alright, continue to talk to her and gain her confidence. If she absolutely refuses treatment, do not proceed. If necessary, emergency services can be called to provide assistance.

Special considerations

There may be times when it will be difficult to communicate with a casualty. Remain confident and caring.

◆ casualty who has difficulty hearing—it may be helpful to have someone use sign language for you. Make sure the casualty can see your face when you speak to help them to read your lips.

◆ casualty who speaks a foreign language—an interpreter may be required.

◆ visually impaired casualty—it is important to explain the care you are providing so she can understand what is happening around her.

◆ children—it is always a good idea for the parents to be present to help comfort the child. It is important that the parents remain calm while around the child. Bring yourself down to the child's eye level, so as not to frighten them.

Principles of communication

Though each situation is different, the following general guidelines help improve communication.

1

Focus   Maintain your attention on the casualty. Position yourself at eye level and maintain eye contact. The casualty will understand that you are truly concerned for her welfare.

Safe Zone   For your own protection, maintain a safe distance from the casualty. The casualty may feel threatened if you enter her "personal space", especially in a highly charged environment. Generally, the safe zone is about one meter (2-3 ft) from the casualty.

Develop contact with the casualty   Address the casualty by name to convey respect. Speak slowly and calmly, use appropriate terminology and do not raise your voice unless the casualty has a hearing problem or you are in a loud environment.

Tell the truth   Don't hide facts or lie about what you are doing. When asked a question always answer truthfully. Use your discretion to limit unnecessary details when appropriate (e.g. when it would needlessly upset the casualty or family).

Terminology   Refrain from using medical terminology when communicating with the casualty or bystanders. Explanations and answers must be clear, concise and easily understood.

Body Language   Refrain from using body language that could be perceived as threatening or aggressive. It is also wise to evaluate the patient's own body language to get an idea of what they might do.

Listen   When a casualty is speaking to you, listen, and try to understand what she is saying. Some casualties will give you clues to the underlying problem, but will not say directly what is truly bothering them. When you ask a question, allow her to answer.

1

Professionalism   Always maintain your professionalism. Explain everything you are doing and why. If what you are doing may be painful, let the casualty know so she is not surprised. When a casualty is speaking to you, listen and respond appropriately.

Politeness   Always assume that the casualty understands what you are saying and doing, especially if she is unconscious or if she does not speak English. Refrain from making inappropriate remarks. An unresponsive casualty may not be able to speak, but may be able to hear. Always consider the casualty's comfort and privacy.

Help at the emergency scene

As a first aider, the first thing you do when you arrive at an emergency scene is take charge of the situation. You stay in charge until you hand control of the scene over to more qualified people. While in charge, many other people may offer to help.

Ten ways a bystander can help

1. Make the area safe.
2. Find all the casualties.
3. Find a first aid kit.
4. Control the crowd.
5. Call for medical help.
6. Help give first aid, under your direction.
7. Gather and protect the casualty's belongings.
8. Take notes.
9. Reassure the casualty's relatives.
10. Lead the paramedics to the scene of the emergency.

Other first aiders

If another first aider arrives on the scene she should tell the first aider in charge that she is trained in first aid and ask if she can help. If someone arrives on the scene and jumps right in, tell that person you are in charge, and ask if she wants to help you.

If you feel another first aider at the scene is more qualified to handle the situation, ask that person to take control. On the other hand, the most qualified person does not need to be in control. The initial first

1

aider at the scene takes charge and stays in charge until she decides to hand over control.

Bystanders

Emergency scenes attract a lot of attention and there may be many people standing around watching. To give the casualty the safest care possible, only the people really needed should be at the scene.

These include:

◆ relatives and close friends of the casualty

◆ any bystanders you ask to stay on the scene to help you

Everyone else should be asked to leave the scene. If needed, have a bystander control the crowd.

Emergency Medical Services (EMS) personnel

Paramedics, police officers and fire fighters are known as EMS personnel. It is their job to respond to an emergency. They are highly trained and will take charge of the scene as soon as they arrive.

Expect them to ask direct questions about the scene, the casualty and your involvement. Tell them you are a first aider, give the history of the scene and the condition of the casualty and follow their instructions. In some situations, you may be asked to continue to care for the casualty.

Other authorities—hydro, telephone, municipal personnel, etc.

Other authorities may be called to the scene (e.g. electrical utility personnel). At an emergency scene, these

1

authorities have a defined role that may not include first aid. Identify yourself, give the history of the scene and ensure the casualty's care is maintained.

Other authorities may arrive by chance. If required, use these people and their equipment to help manage the scene. They may have a radio or portable telephone to call for help. They can direct traffic, control any crowd or help give first aid. Commercial vehicles are often equipped with a first aid kit—this is a good source of first aid supplies if you do not have a kit with you.

Off-duty doctors, nurses and other health professionals

Health professionals are another valuable source of help at an emergency scene. If someone identifies herself as a health professional and asks whether she can help, tell her you are a first aider and that you are in charge of the situation. If the health professional has training and experience in managing the type of illness or injury present, ask for her opinion and advice (do this where the casualty cannot hear you). Make sure that whatever care is given makes sense to you and is best for the casualty.

Handing over control of a scene

When you are in charge of an emergency, you are responsible for the care of the casualty. At some point, you will hand control of the scene over to either another first aider, medical help or to the casualty herself. When deciding to hand over control of the scene, be sure that this is the best course of action for the casualty. Handing control back to the casualty is appropriate when injuries are minor and the casualty can manage without further help.

When handing the scene over to someone other than the casualty, describe the complete history of the incident and

1

pass along any notes you have taken. Be sure to include:

- ◆ your name

- ◆ the time you arrived

- ◆ the history of the illness or injury

- ◆ what first aid has been given

- ◆ any changes in the casualty's condition since you took charge

Medical Help

As a first aider, you are not trained to diagnose the nature and extent of an injury or illness; a medical doctor has the training to do this. As a rule, make sure the casualty receives medical care following first aid. For minor injuries this may not be necessary. In first aid, medical care is called **medical help**.

Medical help is either given by a medical doctor or under the supervision of a medical doctor. Paramedics give medical help because they work under the supervision of medical doctors. Medical help is given in hospitals but it can also be given at the emergency scene or on the way to a medical facility.

Sometimes the need for medical help is urgent and calling for medical help right away is necessary to save the casualty's life. An example might be a car collision where those involved are severely injured. Getting casualties to a hospital where doctors can fully assesss injuries and provide medical care will save the casualty.

1

The Golden Hour

When there are severe, life-threatening injuries, doctors, paramedics and first aiders refer to the **golden hour**. The golden hour is the first hour after the casualty was injured. This time is "golden" because if she makes it to a hospital operating room within this hour, chances of survival are "greatly increased." After one hour, survival rates drop very quickly.

In an emergency there is no time to spare. The sooner the first aider calls for medical help, the better the chances are that the casualty will survive.

Call an ambulance or drive the casualty to the hospital?

Always call an ambulance if you can. Only transport the casualty to medical help yourself if that is the only possible way to get medical help. An ambulance or other rescue vehicle is well-equipped and the casualty can begin receiving medical help as soon as it arrives.

The Good Samaritan principles only protect you when giving care at the scene of the emergency, or while transporting the casualty when this is needed to save the casualty's life and medical help is not available.

The hospital versus the doctor's office

If you call an ambulance to an emergency scene, the paramedics will decide where to take the casualty.

If you or someone else is going to take the casualty to medical help always go to the emergency department of a hospital. You may go to a medical clinic if the situation is not urgent or there is no hospital nearby. As a rule, clinics are not equipped to manage an emergency situation.

Deciding to leave an unresponsive casualty to call medical help

Answer the questions below to help you decide whether you should leave the casualty to get medical help if you are alone.

start here

Is medical help nearby? (meaning, can you get to a phone, call, and return within 3 minutes?)

NO → Stay with the casualty and give life-saving first aid. Once the casualty's life is out of immediate danger, decide whether to go—this is a judgement call.

YES

Can you carry the casualty while going to the phone?

NO → If the unresponsive casualty is an adult, go for medical help. If you will be out of sight of the casualty, turn her into the recovery position before leaving.

If the unresponsive casualty is a child or infant, assess the ABCs. If he is not breathing perform 2 minutes of CPR before leaving to call for help.

YES

Go to call medical help, carrying the casualty with you.

When you return from calling for medical help, start first aid with the primary survey—assessing and giving first aid for the ABCs.

You need to judge the situation, weigh the odds and do your best given your training and experience. Don't make any decision too quickly—also consider your own safety. Whatever you do, keep the risk to yourself as low as possible.

1

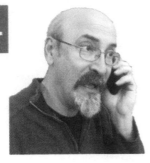

How to get medical help

Medical help is organized under a community's **Emergency Medical Services** (EMS) system. The EMS system is made up of many parts, including ambulance services, hospital emergency departments, doctors, paramedics and fire fighters. As a first aider, you are also an important part of the community EMS system. It is your role to recognize an emergency, give first aid and call for help. Without first aiders and bystanders, the other parts of the EMS system would not be able to respond quickly to emergencies.

To be an effective first aider, you have to know how to get medical help quickly. Know the EMS telephone number for your community (often 9-1-1). If you are outside of your community, the EMS phone number(s) is listed in the first few pages of the telephone book. When you call, follow the dispatcher's instructions. Don't hang up until you are told to, or the dispatcher hangs up first.

Sending a bystander for medical help

If there is a bystander at the scene, it's best to send her to call for medical help. This lets you stay at the scene and give first aid.

Tell the bystander:

◆ to call an ambulance—give her the phone number

◆ to tell the dispatcher what's wrong with the casualty—describe signs and symptoms—do not diagnose

◆ to give the dispatcher the location of the emergency

◆ to report back to you—this way you know the call for medical help has been made

If possible, always send someone out to meet the ambulance. Leading the paramedics to the emergency scene saves a lot of time.

Injuries and illness

1

Injuries

When something from outside the body damages tissues, the damaged area is called an injury. How serious an injury is depends on:

◆ what tissues are injured—an injury to a vital organ, or tissues of a vital system, like the nervous system, is serious

◆ how bad the injury is—for instance, a bone broken in half may not be as serious as the same bone shattered into many pieces

◆ how much tissue is injured—a burned hand may be more serious than a burned finger

Injuries and energy

Injuries result from too much energy being applied to the body. For instance:

◆ a thermal burn is caused by too much heat energy

◆ an acid burn is caused by too much chemical energy

◆ snowblindness is caused by too much light energy

◆ a broken bone is caused by too much mechanical energy

◆ a stopped heart from an electric shock is caused by too much electrical energy

The body can take a certain amount of energy without being injured. But too much of any sort of energy will cause injury. Three factors determine whether an injury will occur. They are:

◆ how intense the energy was

◆ how long the energy was applied to the body

◆ what part of the body the energy was applied to

Most injuries are caused either by something hitting the body or the body hitting something—this is mechanical energy. When something moves, it has mechanical energy. How much mechanical energy something has depends on how fast it is moving and how much it weighs.

Something moving slowly, like a person walking, has less mechanical energy than something the same weight that is moving fast, like a person skiing down a hill. Also, the heavier something is, the more energy it has when it is moving at a given speed. Getting hit by a baseball hurts more than getting hit by a small stone—the baseball is heavier and has more energy—that's why it hurts more.

1

The closer an injury is to vital organs, the more serious the injury is. A broken rib can be more serious than a broken arm because the broken rib could injure a lung and affect breathing.

Mechanism of injury

Every injury has an exact cause. For example, in a car crash, the exact cause is not the the car skidding off the road, but the driver's head hitting the steering wheel. From the moment you arrive at an emergency scene, look for the causes of any injuries. Try to answer these questions:

◆ what happened to the casualty's body to cause the injury?

◆ how much force was involved?

◆ what parts of the body are involved?

The answers to these questions lead to the **mechanism of injury**, which is one of the first aider's most valuable tools. If you understand the mechanism of injury in an emergency situation, you are able to predict what injuries may be present,

Mechanisms of injury that require an ambulance right away

◆ a free fall from more than 6.5 metres (20 feet)

◆ a vehicle collision that shows signs of a severe impact (such as major vehicle damage)

◆ severe damage to the inside of the vehicle that looks as if it was caused by impact with the casualty, like a bent steering wheel or a broken windshield

◆ casualty was thrown from the vehicle

◆ the vehicle rolled over

◆ casualty was struck by a vehicle moving at 30 km/h or more

◆ severe crush injuries

When any of these mechanisms of injury are apparent, call an ambulance as soon as you can; you don't need any more information to make your decision.

1

and what injuries are not likely. If you see that a lot of force or energy was involved, you know right away the person needs an ambulance. Doctors have a list of mechanisms of injury that automatically calls for urgent medical help—these are listed on the opposite page. If you recognize one of these mechanisms of injury, you will know that the casualty needs urgent medical help—call an ambulance right away.

Illness

We often think of first aid in the context of injuries only. But when someone becomes very sick, the result can be a medical emergency in which first aid can save a life.

Some illnesses, like heart attacks or strokes come on very fast. Other illnesses progress more slowly and it can be hard to decide exactly when you have a medical problem that calls for a doctor's attention. Get medical help when any of the following is present:

- ◆ sudden severe pain in any part of the body
- ◆ sudden changes in vision, headache or dizziness
- ◆ severe or persistent diarrhea or vomiting
- ◆ persistent high temperature
- ◆ changes in level of consciousness
- ◆ skin rash of unknown origin
- ◆ repeated fainting
- ◆ obvious depression, suicide threats or attempts
- ◆ whenever you are very worried about yourself or someone in your care

1

If the casualty is an infant, the following are also reasons to get medical help (in addition to the reasons above):

◆ the baby has had a seizure

◆ the baby is blue or very pale

◆ you think the baby is having trouble breathing

◆ the baby cries a lot, or won't stop crying

History, signs and symptoms

Before you can give first aid, you need to assess the casualty to find out what is wrong. All your first aid actions are the result of what you find out in your assessments. History, symptoms and signs are the three ways you get information about a casualty.

History

History is all the information about the emergency situation and the condition of the casualty. You get this information by looking at the scene, talking to witnesses and to the casualty. The history answers the question, "What happened?" For more about the history of the emergency, see page 46.

Signs

Signs are conditions of the casualty you can see, hear, feel and smell such as bleeding or pale skin. You may see the signs of injury or illness immediately, or you may discover them while examining the casualty.

Symptoms

Symptoms are sensations such as pain or dizziness that the casualty feels and may be able to describe. You cannot

1

discover symptoms on your own—the casualty must somehow communicate them to you.

Using history, signs and symptoms

As soon as you arrive on the scene, you are gathering information about the history of the incident, and looking for signs and symptoms. The table below gives examples of the things you may find at an emergency scene that can help you assess the casualty.

Using your first aid knowledge, the signs, symptoms and history at the scene, you will decide what actions to take.

Vital signs

The casualty's temperature, pulse, respiration and level of consciousness are called vital signs. These signs show the basic condition of the casualty—if these signs are normal, the casualty is in pretty good shape. If any of these signs are abnormal, you should be concerned and look further for the reason. The vital signs are discussed in more detail in Chapter 2.

Examples of history, signs and symptoms	
things that can be part of the history	the condition of a vehicle, what bystanders tell you, what the casualty tells you about what happened, objects and substances at the scene, the time of day
signs you can see	blood, deformity, bruising, unequal pupils, painful expression, sweating, wounds, unusual chest movement, skin colour, swelling, foreign bodies, vomit, incontinence
signs you can hear	noisy or distressed breathing, groans, sucking wounds (chest injury), bones scraping together, quality of speech
signs you can feel	dampness, skin temperature, swelling, deformity
signs you can smell	casualty's breath (fruity breath or alcohol), vomit, incontinence, gas fumes, burning, solvents or glue
symptoms the casualty may tell you about	pain, fear, heat, cold, loss of normal movement, loss of sensation, numbness, tingling sensation, thirst, nausea, faintness, stiffness, feeling faint, weakness, memory loss, dizziness, sensation of a broken bone

1

Stress management in emergency situations

First aiders may experience a certain level of stress as a result of the assistance they provide. Stress is the body's normal reaction to physical and psychological events. It can be seen in certain attitudes and behaviors in both casualties and first aiders. It is a biological response and may be reflected in:

◆ an increase in heart rate

◆ an increase in blood pressure

◆ an increase in blood sugar

◆ dilation of the bronchi and pupils

Possible reactions of casualties

Casualties may react to stressors in different ways and first aiders must observe and adjust to such reactions which can include:

◆ denial—the casualty may deny the seriousness of the situation and refuse assistance

◆ resignation—the casualty may be resigned to dying even if his life does not seem to be in danger and doesn't want to make any effort to do what is needed

◆ aggressiveness—the casualty may be hostile

◆ assertive—the casualty is positive, cooperative and may even want to take charge of his or her own care including directing the first aiders

Possible reactions of first aiders

The first aider's reaction time, thinking and efficiency are significantly affected in an emergency situation.

The first aider's response may be expressed in any of the following ways:

physical symptoms—uncontrollable trembling or sudden nausea

general disorganization —feels overwhelmed and may forget important steps or try to do everything all at once

denial—denies the seriousness of the situation and that additional help may be needed

resignation—comes to the conclusion that nothing can be done; it's too late

tunnel effect—the first aider no longer perceives what is going on around him; sees only what is directly related to his source of stress

slowing of time—minutes seem like hours, panic may start to take over especially if waiting for additional help

highly motivated—positive attitude and desire to do whatever he can; usually able to control the stress

Stress Management

Managing stress in an emergency situation can make a significant difference in the quality of first aid provided. Appropriate mental preparation and regular first aid skill practice can help first aiders react effectively when faced with an emergency situation. The negative impact of stress can be reduced by understanding it and taking measures to try and overcome it. After serious incidents, it is important for first aiders to process their emotions. When faced with a highly stressful situation some first aiders may experience prolonged effects of stress and they should seek medical assistance.

Information adapted from the Quebec CSST first aid book

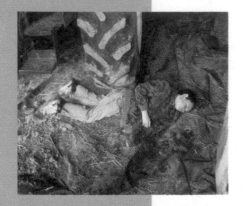

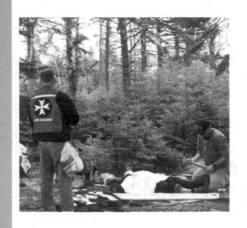

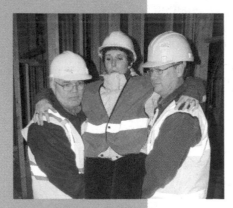

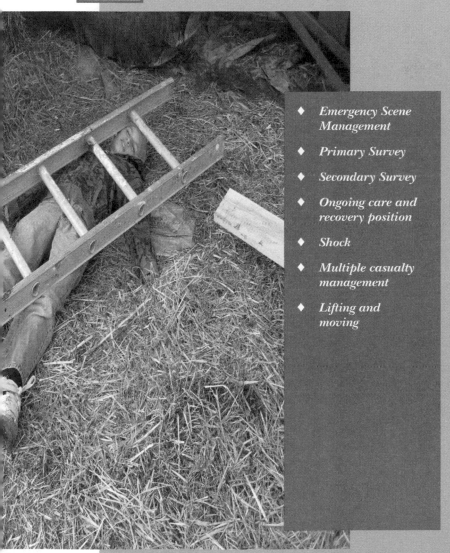

- ◆ *Emergency Scene Management*
- ◆ *Primary Survey*
- ◆ *Secondary Survey*
- ◆ *Ongoing care and recovery position*
- ◆ *Shock*
- ◆ *Multiple casualty management*
- ◆ *Lifting and moving*

Introduction

2

Imagine a busy restaurant at lunchtime—people eating quickly and servers hurrying to get them on their way as fast as possible. Suddenly there is a commotion and you see a woman lying on the ground. What happens now?

Emergency scenes like this usually begin with a lot of confusion as people realize there is an emergency unfolding in front of them—no one knows what to do first, who should be in charge or how they can help. In this situation, the first aider needs to follow a sequence of actions that ensures safe and appropriate first aid is given and everyone's safety is protected. St. John Ambulance first aiders use **emergency scene management** (called ESM for short) to do this.

ESM has four steps:

Emergency scene management is the sequence of actions you should follow to ensure safe and appropriate first aid is given.

◆ *scene survey*—during the scene survey you take control of the scene, find out what happened and make sure the area is safe before assessing the casualty

◆ *primary survey*—during the primary survey you quickly assess the casualty for life-threatening injuries or illnesses and give life-saving first aid

◆ *secondary survey*—the secondary survey is a step-by-step way of gathering information to form a complete picture of the casualty's overall condition

◆ *ongoing casualty care*—during ongoing casualty care you continue to monitor the casualty's condition until medical help takes over

These steps are always done in the order above, though sometimes you don't do the secondary survey. The pages that follow take you through the steps of ESM in detail.

Scene survey

Every emergency scene is different, so the order of the steps of the scene survey will change depending on the situation. As much as possible, however, try to follow the order below.

1   Take charge of the situation

If you're the first first aider on the scene, take charge. If someone is already in charge, ask if you can help. If there is any chance the casualty could have a head or spinal injury, tell the casualty not to move.

2   Call out for help to attract bystanders

You can always use some help in an emergency situation—call out to attract the attention of any bystanders. Do this at any time if you need more help. See Chapter 1 for a list of ten things a bystander can help with.

3   Assess hazards and make the area safe

An emergency scene can be a dangerous place. Look for anything that might be hazardous to the casualty, bystanders or yourself. If there are any hazards, do what you must to make the area safe—bystanders can help you with this. Put on disposable gloves, if possible, to protect yourself as you continue to provide first aid.

4   Find out the history of the emergency, how many casualties there are and the mechanism(s) of injury

By looking at the scene, try to piece together what happened to cause the emergency situation. Look around for all possible casualties and count how many there are. For each casualty, note the mechanism of injury and consider whether there could be a head or spinal injury.

2

5   Identify yourself as a first aider and offer to help

You can only touch someone if you have consent to do so. Before touching the casualty, ask for permission to help. If there is no response, you have implied consent. There is more about consent in Chapter 1.

6   Assess responsiveness

If the casualty responds to you by opening her eyes and speaking, she is conscious. If the casualty's eyes are closed and she is not speaking, tell her, "Open your eyes" while gently tapping her shoulders. Assess how well she responds. If she responds by opening her eyes, or speaking to you, continue with the primary survey. If she does not respond, send for medical help. For more information on when to go for help if you are alone, see Chapter 1.

Next, start the primary survey

By the end of the scene survey, you have begun controlling the scene, have permission to give first aid to the casualty and know whether the casualty is responsive. Next, focus your full attention on the casualty and do the primary survey.

Primary survey

During the primary survey you find out if the casualty has any life-threatening conditions and you give life-saving first aid. The primary survey focuses on the ABCs—airway, breathing and circulation. The exact techniques you use depend on the condition of the casualty. For instance, if the casualty is conscious and talking, you know she has an open airway and is breathing.

How to turn a casualty face up

You should give first aid in the position in which the casualty is found as much as possible. But sometimes you have to turn a casualty over to assess for life-threatening injuries or to give life-saving first aid.

2

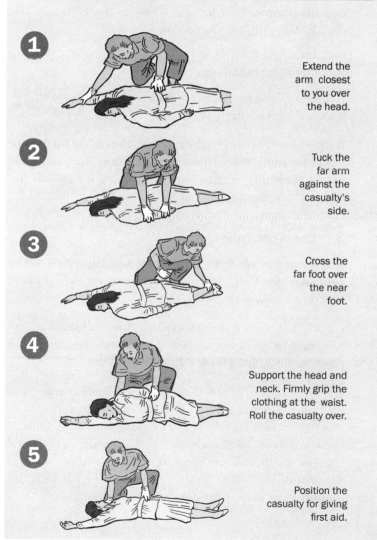

1 Extend the arm closest to you over the head.

2 Tuck the far arm against the casualty's side.

3 Cross the far foot over the near foot.

4 Support the head and neck. Firmly grip the clothing at the waist. Roll the casualty over.

5 Position the casualty for giving first aid.

The primary survey picks up from where the scene survey ends.

2

1   Check the airway

If the casualty is responsive, check the airway by asking a question and seeing how well the casualty can speak. If the casualty is unresponsive the airway may not be open. Use the head-tilt chin-lift to open the airway.

2   Check for breathing

If the casualty is conscious, check for effective breathing by asking if her breathing is okay.

If the casualty is unconscious, check breathing for at least 5 and no more than 10 seconds. If she is not breathing, or not breathing normally (gasping), begin CPR starting with compressions (see Chapter 4).

3   Check circulation

If there is any obvious, severe bleeding, give first aid to control it (see Chapter 5). Bleeding is severe when blood spurts or flows freely from a wound.

Check for shock by assessing skin condition and temperature. If severe bleeding is present or there are signs of shock, send for medical help right away.

If you suspect injuries, do a **rapid body survey** to check for hidden, severe, external bleeding, for signs of severe, internal bleeding and obvious fractures. Quickly run the flats of your hands over the body looking for blood that is hidden from view and for pain or obvious deformity that may indicate serious injury. Expose painful areas to look for signs of internal bleeding.

When doing a rapid body survey:

◆ don't move the casualty unless there is danger

◆ if you can, stay on one side of the casualty. If you must get to the other side, walk around the casualty—never step over a casualty

2

The rapid body survey should take 30 seconds or less.

Provide first aid for life-threatening situations.

◆ Maintain an open airway by placing the unresponsive breathing casualty into the recovery position

◆ Provide CPR if the unresponsive casualty is not breathing or not breathing normally (gasping)

◆ Control severe bleeding

◆ Provide support for obvious fractures

◆ Give first aid for shock by providing first aid for life-threatening injuries and maintaining the casualty's body temperature

Evaluate the situation and decide whether to do a secondary survey

Whether you do a secondary survey depends on the situation. Do a secondary survey if:

◆ the casualty has more than one injury

◆ medical help will be delayed more than 20 minutes

◆ medical help is not coming to the scene and you have to transport the casualty

If you do not do a secondary survey, steady and support any injuries found and give ongoing casualty care (see page 60).

2

Secondary survey

The secondary survey follows the primary survey and any life-saving first aid you had to give. It is a step-by-step way of gathering information to form a complete picture of the condition of the casualty. You are looking for injuries or illnesses that were not revealed in the primary survey, but could benefit from first aid. Only do a complete secondary survey if there is more than one injury, medical help will be delayed more than about 20 minutes, or you have to transport the casualty.

The secondary survey has four steps:

◆ the history

◆ the vital signs

◆ the head-to-toe examination

◆ first aid for injuries and illnesses found

Do not examine for unlikely injuries. For instance, if the casualty cut his hand with a knife while preparing food, there is no need to examine for injuries to the legs. Use the history of the situation and the signs and symptoms of the casualty to decide how much of the head-to-toe examination you need to do. When it is obvious only one part of the body is affected, and the person has no other complaints, a complete head-to-toe examination is not needed.

History

When taking a complete history you are trying to find out everything that could be important about the casualty and the situation. This information can help you give the best first aid possible, and passing this information on may be helpful to others who care for the casualty.

2

If the casualty is fully conscious, ask her questions directly. If the casualty is unconscious or confused, ask friends, relatives and bystanders about her and the situation.

A simple way to take a complete history of the casualty is to remember the word **SAMPLE**. Each letter stands for a part of the history, as follows:

S = *symptoms.* Symptoms are sensations the casualty feels such as pain, nausea, etc. If the casualty is conscious, ask her what she is feeling. If she is unconscious, ask bystanders if she complained of any symptoms before losing consciousness.

A = *allergies.* If the casualty is conscious, ask her if she has any allergies. Particularly important here are allergies to medications.

M = *medications.* Ask if the casualty has taken any medication in the past 24 hours. Does she regularly take medication she may NOT have taken today?

P = *past or present medical history.* Ask about the casualty's medical history and whether there is anything that could be related to the current injury or illness. Check for a medical alert device.

L = *last meal.* Find out when the casualty ate her last meal. This may be important information for medical help.

E = *events leading to the incident.* Ask how the incident happened. Consider how the casualty's body was affected—this will help you find all injuries.

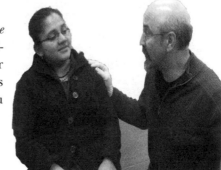

2

Vital signs

The **four vital signs** show the basic condition of the casualty. These are:

◆ level of consciousness (LOC)

◆ breathing

◆ pulse

◆ skin condition and temperature

Any change in a casualty's vital signs can indicate a serious change in condition. Once you have assessed (or "taken") the vital signs, monitor them closely— every few minutes, or whenever you think the casualty's condition may have changed.

 Taking the vital signs

1   Assess level of consciousness (LOC).

Use the Modified Glasgow Coma Scale to assess LOC—see page 50.

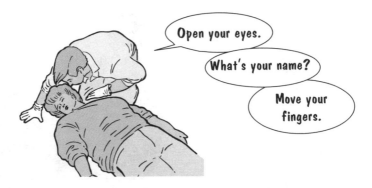

2   Assess breathing—see page 51.

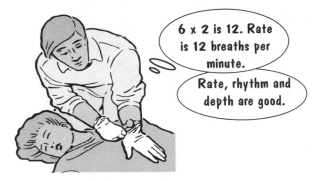

3   Assess the pulse—see page 52.

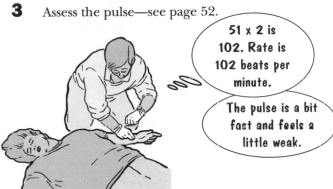

4   Assess skin condition and temperature—see page 53.

Reassess the vital signs every few minutes or when you think the casualty's condition has changed. Write down what you find using a form like the one shown on page 371, if you have one. Once you have taken the vital signs, do a head-to-toe examination of the casualty.

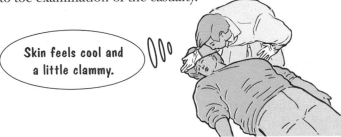

Vital signs – How to assess level of consciousness (LOC)

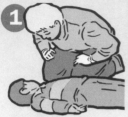 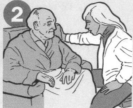 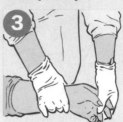

Check eye opening response. If the casualty's eyes are open, he is conscious. If the casualty's eyes are not open, say, "Open your eyes." If the casualty's eyes still don't open, pinch the skin on the forearm to see if mild pain causes the eyes to open.

Check verbal response. Ask questions and listen to how well the casualty can speak. Is the casualty:

◆ oriented and alert?

◆ confused and not making sense?

◆ not able to speak?

Check motor response. How well can the casualty move? Ask him to move part of his body. If there is no response, squeeze the thumbnail to cause mild pain and see if that causes the casualty to move.

Record the LOC

1. Eye opening response
    - ☐ eyes open
    - ☑ eyes open to speech or pain
    - ☐ eyes don't open

2. Verbal response
    - ☐ oriented and alert
    - ☐ confused, doesn't make sense
    - ☑ no speech

3. Motor response
    - ☑ obeys commands
    - ☐ moves to pain
    - ☐ no movement

This casualty's LOC would be described as, "Eyes open to speech, no verbal response, obeys commands."

This method of assessing LOC is called the Modified Glasgow Coma Scale.

Causing pain

Note any pain reactions you see as you do the primary and secondary surveys. Use these to assess LOC.

Casualty's response

Some conditions may affect the casualty's ability to respond but should not affect the LOC rating. For instance:

◆ an eye injury or swelling around the eyes will affect eye opening response

◆ a throat injury, speech disability or a language barrier may affect verbal response

◆ paralysis will affect motor response—if you suspect paralysis, check motor response by asking the casualty to blink his eyes

Vital signs – How to assess breathing

In the primary survey you performed an initial breathing check.

In the secondary survey, you assess breathing rate, rhythm and depth, as these are important indictors of a person's state of health. These signs give early warning of physical changes and of life-threatening conditions. Breathing:

◆ rate refers to how many breaths the person takes in one minute—it is assessed as "breaths per minute."

◆ rhythm refers to how regular the intervals between breaths are—rhythm is assessed as either "regular" or "irregular."

◆ depth refers to how deeply the person is breathing—depth is assessed as "shallow," "normal" or "deep." There is more on breathing rate, rhythm and depth starting on page 95.

If the casualty is conscious

Look at the casualty's chest and abdomen and ask about her breathing. Listen not only to what the casualty says, but also, to how well she is able to say it.

Assess breathing rate, rhythm and depth as for the unconscious casualty.

If the casualty is unconscious

Place a hand on the chest and assess breathing rate, rhythm and depth. Look for other signs of severe breathing difficulties also—see page 97.

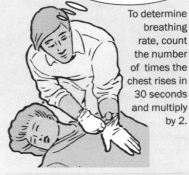

6 x 2 is 12. Rate is 12 breaths per minute.

To determine breathing rate, count the number of times the chest rises in 30 seconds and multiply by 2.

Record the breathing assessment

1. Breathing rate
   - ☐ below the normal range
   - ☑ within the normal range
   - ☐ above the normal range

2. Breathing rhythm
   - ☑ regular intervals between breaths
   - ☐ irregular intervals between breaths

3. Breathing depth
   - ☐ shallow breathing
   - ☑ normal
   - ☐ deep breathing

4. Other comments on breathing

   ☐

Breathing rates – breaths per minute

age group	range of normal rates	too slow	too fast
infant	30 to 50	below 25	above 60
child	20 to 30	below 15	above 40
adult	10 to 20	below 10	above 30

2

Vital signs – How to take the pulse

For an adult or child casualty, take the pulse at the wrist and/or neck. For an infant casualty, take the pulse on the inside of the upper arm.

Taking an adult's or child's pulse

The radial pulse is commonly used for an adult or child casualty. The radial pulse is located at the base of the thumb on either wrist.

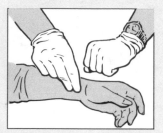

If you can't find the radial pulse, check the carotid pulse on either side of the neck. Feel for a pulse on the side closest to you. Do not feel or compress both sides at the same time.

Slide two fingers into the groove of the neck just down from the Adam's apple. Press gently to detect the pulse.

Taking an infant's pulse

The best place to take the pulse of an infant is on the upper arm. This pulse is called the brachial pulse. You find it halfway down the inside of the upper arm, between the large muscle of the arm and the bone.

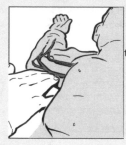

Press gently to feel the pulse. Count the number of heartbeats in 30 seconds and multiply by 2.

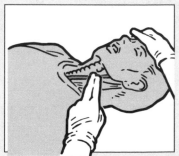

Normal pulse rates

age	rate (heartbeats per min.)
adult	60-80
child	80-150
infant	120-150

Never use your thumb to take the pulse—it has a pulse of its own, and you will feel your own pulse instead of the casualty's.

2

Vital signs – How to assess skin condition and temperature

The condition and temperature of the skin change when there is shock. By assessing the skin, you are checking for shock. The signs and symptoms of shock are listed on page 67.

To assess skin condition, look for:

◆ the skin colour

– is the skin pale, reddish or bluish?

◆ the presence of sweating

– is the skin wet or clammy?

To assess skin temperature, place the back of your hand on the forehead, neck or cheek. If the skin is pale and cool, or pale, cool and clammy, shock is present.

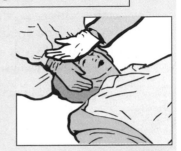

Head-to-toe examination

Use the head-to-toe examination to find and examine other injuries and illnesses that may need first aid.

Fully conscious casualty

If the casualty is fully conscious:

◆ ask him where it hurts and examine that area first. If he tells you there are two or more areas that hurt, ask, "Which one is bothering you most?"

◆ ask if anything else is wrong and make sure there are no injuries that are masked by pain, numbness or drugs

As you do the head-to-toe examination, talk to the casualty even if he is unconscious. Although an unconscious casualty cannot respond to you, he may still be able to hear you. By telling the casualty what you are doing, he will be reassured whether he is fully conscious or just barely able to understand you. Ask the conscious casualty his name and use it when speaking to him.

2

If you must get to the other side, walk around the casualty—never step over a casualty.

Don't comment on "how bad" an injury is and don't tell the casualty what you think the problem might be—only a medical doctor can properly diagnose an illness or injury. Instead, tell the casualty what you are going to do, what you are doing, and why you are doing it. If the casualty asks you specific questions about his injuries, tell him what you see and that a doctor will determine the extent of the injury or illness.

Head-to-toe examination

1   Examine the head.

◆ check the skull and scalp. Look for bruising, blood and swelling. Feel for bumps, depressions or anything abnormal

◆ check the face. Compare one side to the other. Is one side obviously drooping?

◆ check the eyes—look for any bruising

◆ gently open both eyes and compare the pupils—are they both the same size?

◆ check the lips and mouth—are the lips burned, bleeding or discoloured? Is there an odour on the breath?

◆ open the mouth and look in—is there anything in the mouth the casualty could choke on, like candy, gum, loose dentures or loose teeth? Remove any loose objects

◆ check the ears for blood or clear fluid that may indicate a head injury

◆ check the nose for swelling, blood or clear fluid

2   Check the neck.

◆ look and gently feel for deformities

◆ check for a medical alert necklace

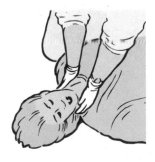

2

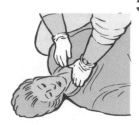

3   Check the collarbones one at a time.

◆ gently run your fingers along the full
   length of the collarbones, feeling for
   deformities

◆ look for signs of injury

4   Check the shoulders, arms and hands.

◆ check one side first, then check the
   other side. If you can't safely reach
   over the casualty, walk around to the
   other side

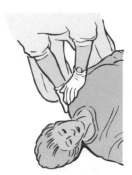

◆ check the shoulder joint

◆ check as much of the shoulder
   blade as you can without moving the
   casualty. Check the full length of the
   arm. Squeeze the hand and check
   each of the fingers

◆ check the colour of the fingernails—
   are they blue? This may be a sign of
   shock

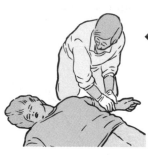

◆ ask the conscious casualty if she has
   feeling in her arm, hand and fingers,
   and if she can move them

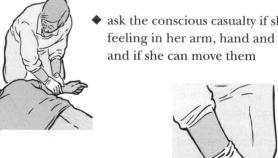

5   Check the chest and under.

◆ watch and feel the chest move—
does it cxpand casily, evenly and
equally on both sides?

◆ feel for wounds and other injuries

◆ ask the conscious casualty to take
a deep breath to see if this causes
any pain

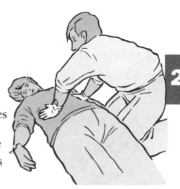

6   Check the abdomen and under.

◆ gently press on the abdomen—does this cause
pain? Is the abdomen tender? Does it feel hard or
stiff?

◆ ask the conscious casualty to pull
in and push out the abdomen —
does this cause any pain?

◆ check as much of the back as
possible without moving the casualty

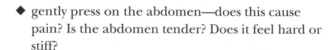

Medical alert information

People who have ongoing medical conditions that need specific treatment often wear or carry medical information in a variety of forms ranging from a bracelet or necklace to tatoos. Sometimes this information is kept in a specially marked container on the top shelf in the person's refrigerator.

These medical alert devices state the condition and perhaps the treatment

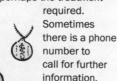

required. Sometimes there is a phone number to call for further information.

When examining an unconscious casualty, look for medical alert information. It could help in your assessment and might warn of allergies or health problems that would make certain first aid or medical procedures dangerous. Tell whomever you hand the casualty over to about the medical alert information.

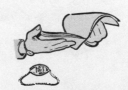

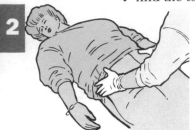

7   Check the pelvis and buttocks.

◆ find the top of the pelvic bones

    ◆ gently squeeze the tops of the pelvic bones towards each other and check whether this causes pain

8   Check the legs, ankles and feet.

◆ look at the legs—is there any obvious deformity? Is one foot turned in or out in an unnatural way? Is one leg shorter than the other?

◆ feel for injuries one leg at a time. With firm pressure, check the upper leg, all around the knee, the front and back of the lower leg and all around the ankle

    ◆ squeeze the foot and each toe and ask the casualty if she can feel your touch

    ◆ ask the conscious casualty if she has feeling in the leg, foot and toes and whether she can move them

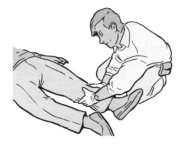

2

Finding injuries during the head-to-toe examination

When a casualty tells you where an injury is, or when you find an injury during the head-to-toe examination, don't stop your examination. Instead, examine the injury just enough to determine the type and severity, then complete the head-to-toe examination. By stopping at one injury, you can forget to examine the rest of the casualty.

If you find a life-threatening injury that was missed in the primary survey, provide the appropriate first aid immediately.

Giving first aid for injuries and illnesses found

To give appropriate first aid, each injury must be carefully examined. You need to have a good look to find out the nature and extent of the tissue damage. The most important part of examining an injury is exposing it. If clothing is in the way, it is best to cut it—trying to take it off may cause you to move the injured part in the process. If clothing is stuck to the injury, don't pull it off—this could cause further tissue damage. Always tell the casualty what item of clothing you are removing and why. And always respect a casualty's privacy when removing clothing.

The most important part of examining an injury is exposing it.

When you have finished the head-to-toe examination, give the appropriate first aid for any injury or illness you have found or suspect. If there is more than one injury or illness, use the priorities for casualties with more than one injury (see chart on page 75) to decide which injury to care for first.

Deciding what first aid to give depends on whether medical help will be coming to the scene, how long it will take to arrive if it is coming and the first aid the casualty needs. If medical help will arrive within 30 minutes it may be best to support the casualty in the position found until medical help arrives. The best first aid depends on the details of the situation.

Ongoing casualty care

Once first aid for injuries and illnesses that are not life threatening has been given, one of three things will happen:

- ◆ you hand over control of the scene to the casualty, or someone else, and end your involvement in the emergency

- ◆ you stay in control of the scene and wait for medical help to take over, or

- ◆ you stay in control of the scene and transport the casualty to medical help (see page 29) on when to do this

When you stay in control of the scene, you should continue giving first aid to keep the casualty in the best possible condition. This first aid is called **ongoing casualty care**. It includes:

- ◆ showing a bystander how to maintain manual support of any injuries, if needed

- ◆ continuing first aid for shock

- ◆ monitoring the casualty's condition, especially ABCs

- ◆ giving nothing by mouth. If the casualty complains of thirst, moisten her lips with a wet cloth

- ◆ recording the casualty's condition, any changes that occur, and the first aid given (sample form on page 371)

- ◆ protecting the casualty's personal belongings

- ◆ handing the casualty over to medical help and reporting on the incident, the casualty's condition and the first aid given

How to put a casualty into the recovery position

This position protects the casualty and also reduces bending and twisting of the spine. This position protects the airway if you must leave the casualty.

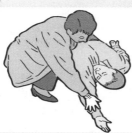

Position the arm closest to you with the arm above the casualty's head.

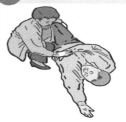

Position the arm furthest from you on the casualty's chest. Bend the far knee.

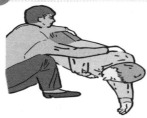

Reach behind the casualty's shoulder and roll to casualty towards you by pulling on the far knee.

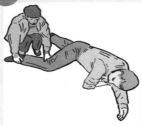

Adjust the position of the arms and leg so the casualty is in a stable position. Place the far arm at 90 degrees to the casualty with the palm down. Place padding behind casualty to prevent him rolling back into a face up position.

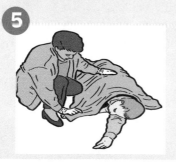

Give ongoing care.

After the handover

2

In first aid, we prepare ourselves to care for an injured or ill person. We don't often think about what happens after the casualty has left our care. Immediately following the handover of the casualty you may have a number of practical details to attend to. These details can include cleaning up after the emergency, correcting any unsafe conditions that caused the injury, or making a report on the incident and your involvement.

Once these practical matters are out of the way, we expect things to "return to normal." However, you will likely find yourself thinking about the situation and the details of what happened while you were involved. Following a stressful event, many people review the details and try to evaluate what they did and how they could have done it better.

The effects of critical incident stress can appear many weeks, months or years after the event.

This reviewing of the events is completely normal and you can expect it to happen. But if thoughts of the incident continue for many weeks, or if they affect your day-to-day life, you may be experiencing the negative effects of **critical incident stress** (CIS).

Critical incident stress is a common reaction to a stressful emergency situation. The effects of CIS can interfere with your daily life—your job, your relationships, your peace of mind. If this happens to you, you need to do something about it, and help is readily available. Start by talking to your family doctor or a doctor at a walk-in clinic. A doctor will understand what you are going through and will suggest a course of action.

How ESM changes when a head or spinal injury is suspected

2

If you suspect a head or spinal injury, protect the head and neck from any movement. Head or neck movement could result in life-long disability or death. Adjust your first aid to this situation as shown below.

1

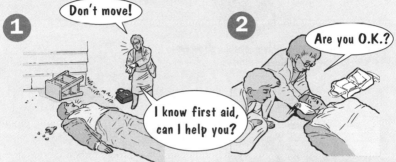

As soon as you see there might be a head or spinal injury, tell the casualty not to move.

2

Once you have consent to help the casualty, steady and support the head and neck. Keep elbows firmly supported on thighs or ground. Then, assess responsiveness.

3

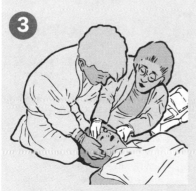

If there is a bystander to help, show her how to support the head and neck so you can continue your assessment.

4

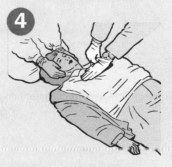

Continue your assessment.

2

5

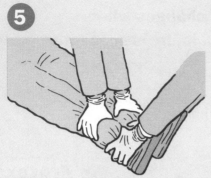

If a second bystander is available, show him how to steady and support the feet to prevent movement.

6

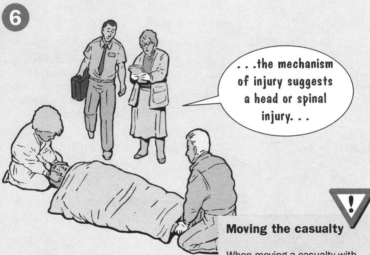

. . .the mechanism of injury suggests a head or spinal injury. . .

Keep the head and neck supported (and the feet if possible) while giving further first aid until handover to medical help, or until the casualty is completely immobilized on a long spine board—see page 282.

Moving the casualty

When moving a casualty with a suspected head or spinal injury, move him as a unit as much as possible. This means rolling the head, trunk and legs together, or lifting the whole body at the same time. Do what you can to prevent movement, including twisting, of the spine.

How to turn a casualty face up

You should give first aid in the position in which the casualty is found as much as possible. But sometimes you have to turn a casualty over to assess for life-threatening injuries or to give life-saving first aid.

Suspected head or spinal injury (multiple first aider)

When you suspect a head or spinal injury, turn the casualty as a unit so the head and spine stay in the same relative position.

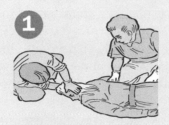

The first aider at the head supports the head—placing the right hand along the right side of the casualty's head and the left hand along the left side.

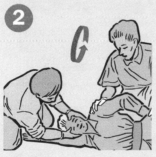

The other first aider extends the casualty's near arm over her head and gets a good grip on the casualty at the shoulder and waist.

At the same time, the two first aiders roll the casualty towards the second first aider.

If extra help is available, have the third first aider support the legs to prevent twisting of the neck and spine. With a fourth, put one first aider at the shoulders and another at the waist.

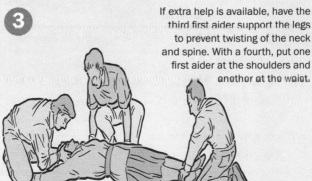

Shock

2

Any injury or illness can be accompanied by shock. Shock is a circulation problem where the body's tissues don't get enough oxygenated blood. This is medical shock—don't confuse it with an electric shock or "being shocked" as in scared or surprised. Medical shock is life-threatening because the brain and other organs cannot function properly. As shock progresses, it leads to unconsciousness and even death. Because there is often shock in an emergency situation, and because it can progress very quickly, always check for shock and assess whether it is serious enough to be a medical emergency by itself. Like safety, shock is one of those things you always have to be thinking about.

Common causes of severe shock	
Cause of shock	**How it causes a circulation problem**
severe bleeding - internal or external (includes major fractures)	not enough blood to fill blood vessels
severe burns	loss of blood plasma (fluid) into tissues—not enough blood to fill blood vessels
crush injuries	loss of blood and blood plasma into tissues—not enough blood to fill blood vessels
heart attack	heart is not strong enough to pump blood effectively
spinal cord or nerve injuries	brain can't control the size of the blood vessels—the blood can't get to the tissues properly
severe allergic reactions	many things can be affected—breathing, heart function, etc.

The table above gives some causes of shock. Severe shock can also result from medical emergencies such as diabetes, epilepsy, infection, poisoning or a drug overdose. Pain, anxiety and fear don't cause shock, but they can help make it worse, or make it progress faster. This is why reassuring a casualty and making her comfortable is so important.

Signs and symptoms of shock

Signs

◆ pale skin at first, turns blue-grey *

◆ blue-purple lips, tongue, earlobes, fingernails

◆ cold and clammy skin

◆ breathing shallow and irregular, fast or gasping for air

◆ changes in level of consciousness

◆ weak, rapid pulse— radial pulse may be absent

Symptoms

◆ restless

◆ anxious

◆ disoriented

◆ confused

◆ afraid

◆ dizzy

◆ thirsty

* For casualties with dark skin, check the inside of the lips– mucous membranes should be pink.

 First aid for shock

The following actions will minimize shock:

1 Give first aid for the injury or illness that caused the shock.

2 Reassure the casualty often.

3 Minimize pain by handling the casualty gently.

4 Loosen tight clothing at the neck, chest and waist.

5 Keep the casualty warm, but do not overheat—use jackets, coats or blankets if you have them.

2

6 Moisten the lips if the casualty complains of thirst. Don't give anything to eat or drink. If medical help is delayed many hours, give small amounts of water or clear fluids to drink—make a note of what was given and when.

7 Place the casualty in the best position for her condition.

8 Continue ongoing casualty care until hand over.

The above first aid for shock also prevents shock from getting worse. Whenever possible, add these steps to any first aid you give—this will minimize shock.

Positioning a casualty in shock

Putting the casualty in the right position can slow the progress of shock and make the casualty more comfortable. The position you use depends on the casualty's condition. The casualty should be as comfortable as possible in the position you use.

No suspected head/spinal injury; fully conscious

Place the casualty on his back. Once the casualty is positioned, cover him to preserve body heat, but do not overheat.

No suspected head/spinal injury; less than fully conscious

Place the casualty in the recovery position (see page 61). When there is decreased level of consciousness, airway and breathing are the priority—the recovery position ensures an open airway.

Suspected head/spinal injury

If you suspect a head or spinal injury, steady and support the casualty in the position found and monitor the ABCs closely. This protects the head and spine from further injury.

As injuries permit

A casualty's injuries may not permit you to put her into the best position. Always think of the casualty's comfort when choosing a position.

Head and spinal injuries

Injuries to the head and spine (especially the neck) are a special concern because they can be life-threatening and/or cause life-long disability. Whenever you suspect a head injury, also suspect a neck injury, and whenever you suspect a neck injury, also suspect a head injury. Because the head and neck are so close to each other, often, when one is injured, so is the other.

In every emergency situation, ask yourself if there is any way there could be a head or neck injury. Do this by looking at:

◆ the mechanism of injury

◆ the position of the casualty

◆ the history of the incident, including:

   ❖ what you are told

   ❖ what you can figure out from looking around the scene

Decreased level of consciousness (LOC)

2

Consciousness means how aware a person is of herself and her surroundings. There is a full range of levels of consciousness, from completely conscious to completely unconscious. Many injuries and illnesses can cause changes in a casualty's level of consciousness. Some examples are:

◆ a breathing emergency

◆ a head injury

◆ shock

◆ a medical condition (epilepsy, diabetes, etc.)

◆ a heart attack

◆ poisoning

◆ alcohol or drug abuse

Unconsciousness may cause a breathing emergency

Semi-consciousness and unconsciousness can cause breathing emergencies because, in an unconscious person, the tongue may fall to the back of the throat and block the airway. Also, saliva and other fluids can pool at the back of the throat. Since an unconscious person loses the reflex to clear fluids in the throat, the fluids block the airway and choke the person.

A progressive loss of consciousness means the casualty's condition is getting worse. Always monitor a casualty's level of consciousness and note any changes.

First aid for unconsciousness

2

1 Start ESM—do a scene survey. Have a bystander call for medical help as soon as unresponsiveness is determined (see page 29 for what to do if you are alone).

2 Do a primary survey.

3 Do a secondary survey if necessary.

4 Turn the casualty into the recovery position, if injuries permit. Give ongoing care.

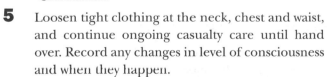

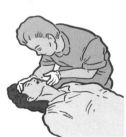

If injuries make it necessary for the casualty to be face up, monitor breathing continuously. If necessary, hold the airway open. Always ensure an open airway.

5 Loosen tight clothing at the neck, chest and waist, and continue ongoing casualty care until hand over. Record any changes in level of consciousness and when they happen.

Decreased consciousness is always an urgent situation. The person can quickly become unconscious, causing a breathing emergency. When you recognize decreased consciousness, get medical help as fast as possible.

If you have to leave to get medical help or you have to give first aid to other casualties, turn the casualty into the recovery position being as careful as you can if there are any injuries.

2

Fainting

Fainting is a loss of consciousness that lasts a very short time—no more than a few minutes. It is caused by a temporary shortage of oxygenated blood to the brain. Some common reasons people faint are:

◆ fear or anxiety

◆ severe pain, injury or illness

◆ underlying medical problem

◆ long periods of standing or sitting

◆ lack of fresh air

◆ the sight of blood

◆ fatigue or hunger

Loss of consciousness is always a serious medical emergency. Do not assume a person has "just fainted" until there is a quick, full recovery and the reason for the fainting is known. If you think there might be a serious reason a person feels faint, or has fainted, get medical help.

Feeling faint or "impending faint"

Sometimes when a person is about to faint, there are warning signs. The person:

◆ is pale

◆ is sweating

◆ feels sick, nauseous, dizzy or unsteady

When a person is about to faint, act quickly.

First aid for an impending faint

1 Place the casualty on her back.

2 Ensure a supply of fresh air—open windows or doors.

3 Loosen tight clothing at the neck, chest and waist.

4 Stay with the casualty until she has fully recovered.

First aid for fainting

A person who has fainted is unconscious. The first aid for fainting is the same as the first aid for unconsciousness (see page 71).

◆ Ensure a supply of fresh air and loosen tight clothing at the neck, chest and waist. Continue ongoing casualty care until hand over.

◆ Make the casualty comfortable as consciousness returns and keep her lying down for 10 to 15 min. Continue to monitor breathing and consciousness.

Recovery from a faint should be quick and complete. If the casualty has recovered, have her get up slowly to prevent another incident. If the casualty is not feeling stronger, stay with her until medical help takes over.

Multiple casualty management (triage)

2

You are travelling alone and arrive at the scene of a car crash—there are at least four casualties. Who do you go to first?

When there are more casualties than first aiders, you need a system to ensure that the casualties get the best treatment without time being wasted on unnecessary things. You need an approach that will help you save as many lives as possible.

The process of making these decisions at an emergency scene where people are injured is called **triage**. In triage, first aiders quickly examine all casualties and place them in order of greatest need for first aid and for transportation. The idea is to do the most good for the greatest number of casualties.

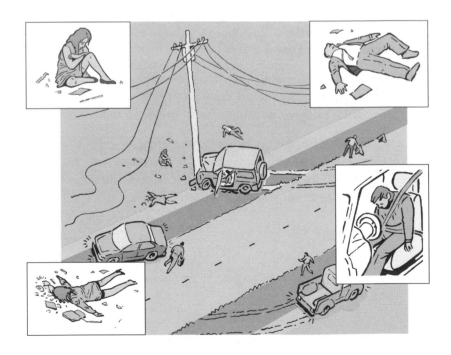

Three levels of priority

The table below shows the priorities for different injuries and conditions. There are three levels of priority:

2

◆ **highest priority**—casualties who need immediate first aid and transportation to medical help

◆ **second priority**—casualties who probably can wait one hour for medical help without risk to their lives

◆ **lowest priority**—casualties who can wait and receive first aid and transportation last, or casualties who are obviously dead

The first aid priorities for injuries

Priority	Condition	Causes
1st – Airway	foreign body blocking airway	choking on food
	tongue or fluids blocking airway	unconscious, lying on back
	swollen airway	allergic reaction, airway infection
2nd – Breathing	injured chest and/or lungs	chest injury, broken ribs
	brain not controlling breathing properly	poisoning, drug overdose, stroke, electric shock
	not enough oxygen reaching blood	not enough oxygen in air, carbon monoxide poisoning
3rd – Circulation	severe bleeding	external bleeding or internal bleeding
	severe shock	bleeding, serious illness, poisoning
Injuries that may affect ABCs or have potential for life-long disability	fractures that could affect breathing	broken ribs, shoulder blade
	fractures—open, severe or multiple bones	broken upper leg, pelvis, crushed arm
	head/spinal injuries	fall from a 6-foot ladder
	critical burns	3rd degree burns to the hands
Minor injuries or obviously dead	minor fractures	broken lower leg, lower arm, hand, finger, etc.
	minor bleeding	bleeding not spurting or free-flowing
	non-critical burns	2nd degree burns to the forearms
	behavioural problems	grief or panic
	obviously dead	obvious massive injuries, no pulse or other signs of circulation

high priority

second priority

low priority

Triage sequence of actions

Triage is a decision-making process. One person should be in charge of the triage process—the most experienced first aider. Stay calm, continually assess the hazards and don't risk your own safety.

1   Begin ESM—start the scene survey. Try to determine how many casualties there are.

2   Go to the nearest casualty, provided it is safe to do so. Assess responsiveness and do a primary survey. Give first aid for life-threatening conditions—only do what you have to do to save the person's life. If the person is obviously dead, don't waste time. Go to the next nearest casualty.

3   Repeat step 2 for each casualty in turn, always going to the next nearest casualty.

4   Once you have done a primary survey on each casualty, decide which casualties have the highest priority, second priority and lowest priority.

5   If there are injuries of the highest priority, and transportation to medical help is available, arrange transportation for those casualties.

6   Do a secondary survey on each casualty, starting with the casualties of the highest priority. Give appropriate first aid—most injuries can simply be steadied and supported.

7   Continue ongoing casualty care for each casualty.

In a multiple casualty situation, you must constantly assess the changing conditions of both the casualties and the situation itself and make changes to the priorities. When medical help arrives, tell the paramedics it is a triage situation and answer their questions.

Lifting and moving

Always try to give necessary first aid where the casualty is found, then wait for the paramedics to move the person. However, there are times when this is not possible.

2

You may have to move a casualty when:

◆ there are life-threatening hazards to yourself or the casualty e.g. danger from fire, explosion, gas or water

◆ essential first aid for wounds or other conditions cannot be given in the casualty's present position or location

◆ the casualty must be transported to a medical facility

If life-threatening hazards make it necessary to move a casualty right away, you may need to use a rescue carry.

In urgent and dangerous situations where casualties are moved with less than ideal support for injuries, the casualty's injuries may be made worse by improper movement and handling. The chance of further injury can be reduced with proper rescue carry techniques.

Always move the casualty the shortest possible distance to safety and to provide essential first aid. Use bystanders to help you and support any injuries the best you can during the move. Keep the risks to the casualty, yourself and others to a minimum.

2

Choose the best method

Moving any casualty from an emergency scene poses dangers to the rescuer as well as the casualty. If the casualty must be moved, select the method that will pose the least risk to the casualty and to yourself. You can be of little help to a casualty if you injure yourself in the rescue.

Lifting techniques and proper body mechanics

Using incorrect body mechanics in lifting or moving a casualty may leave the rescuer suffering muscle strains. Use the following lifting guidelines:

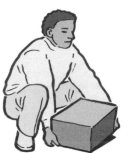

1   Stand close to the object to be lifted.

2   Bend your knees, not your waist.

3   Tilt the object so that you can put one hand under the edge or corner closest to you.

4   Place your other hand under the opposite side or corner, getting a good grip on the object.

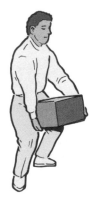

5   Use your leg muscles to lift, and keep your back straight.

6   When turning, turn your feet first; don't twist your body.

When lowering the object, reverse the procedure.

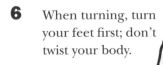

Rescue carries

A rescue carry is an emergency method of moving a casualty over a short distance to safety, shelter or to transportation. Select the type of carry based on the circumstances.

◆ the size and weight of the casualty relative to the rescuer

◆ the number of rescuers available to assist

◆ the type of injury

◆ the distance to move the casualty

Whenever possible, ask one or more bystanders to help you. When help is available:

◆ remain with the casualty

◆ give instructions to the bystanders about what to do and what safety precautions to take

◆ fully coordinate the rescue activities

Because of the risk of aggravating any injuries, only use drag carries in the most extreme cases when there is an immediate threat to life.

Drag carry

This carry is used by the single rescuer to drag a casualty who is either lying on his back or in a sitting position. The drag carry provides maximum protection to the head and neck.

If time permits, tie the casualty's wrists together across her chest before dragging.

1 Stand at the casualty's head facing her feet.

2 Crouch down and ease your hands under the casualty's shoulders. Grasp the clothing on each side. Support the casualty's head between your forearms to stop movement.

3 Drag the casualty backward only as far as necessary for her safety.

As an alternate method, the first aider can use a blanket to support and drag the casualty.

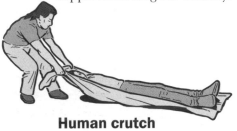

Human crutch

If a leg or foot is injured, help the casualty to walk on his good leg while you give support to the injured side.

1 Take the weight of the casualty's injured side on your shoulders by placing the casualty's arm (on the injured side) around your neck and grasping the wrist firmly.

2 Reach around the casualty's back with your free hand, and grasp his clothing at the waist.

3 Tell the casualty to step off with you, each using the inside foot. This lets you, the rescuer, take the casualty's weight on the injured side.

Chair carry

The chair carry enables two rescuers to carry a conscious or unconscious casualty through narrow passages and up and down stairs. Do not use this carry for casualties with suspected neck or back injuries. Specially designed rescue chairs are available and should be used for this type of carry.

If the casualty is unconscious or helpless:

1 Place an unconscious casualty on a chair by sliding the back of the chair under his legs and buttocks, and along the lower back.

2 Strap his upper body and arms to the back of the chair.

3 Two rescuers carry the chair, one at the front and one at the back. The rescuer at the back crouches and grasps the back of the chair, while the rescuer at the front crouches between the casualty's knees and grasps the front chair legs near the floor.

4 The rescuers walk out-of-step.

Going down stairs

◆ The casualty faces forward

◆ The front rescuer faces the casualty

◆ A third person should act as a guide and support the front rescuer in case he loses his footing

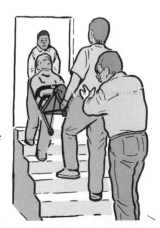

2

Extremities carry

Use the extremities carry when you don't have a chair and you don't suspect fractures of the trunk, head or spine.

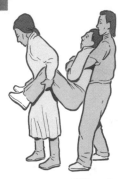

1   One rescuer passes his hands under the casualty's armpits and grasps the casualty's wrists, crossing them over his chest.

2   The second rescuer crouches with her back between the casualty's knees and grasps each leg just above the knee.

3   The rescuers step off on opposite feet— walking out-of-step is smoother for the casualty.

Blanket lift with four bearers

1   Roll the blanket or rug lengthwise for half its width. Position bearers at the head and feet to keep the head, neck and body in line. Place the rolled edge along the casualty's injured side.

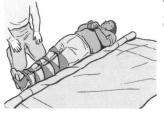

2   Kneel at the casualty's shoulder and position another bearer at the waist to help logroll the casualty onto the uninjured side. Turn the casualty as a unit so the casualty's body is not twisted during the logroll (see page 284 for more on the logroll).

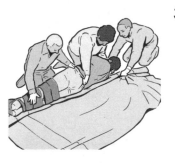

3   Roll the casualty back over the blanket roll to lay face up on the blanket. Unroll the blanket and then roll the edges of the blanket to each side of the casualty. Get ready to lift the casualty—have the bearers grip the rolls at the head and shoulders, and at the hip and legs.

4 Keep the blanket tight as the casualty is lifted and placed on the stretcher.

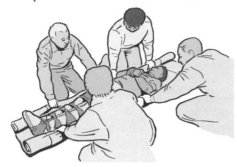

Before using a blanket, test it to ensure that it will carry the casualty's weight.

Do not use this lift if neck or back injuries are suspected.

Stretchers

There may be times when medical help cannot be contacted, or for other reasons, cannot come to the scene. When this happens, transport the casualty to medical help. If the casualty can't walk, or if the injury or illness allows only the most gentle movement, a stretcher should be used.

Commercial stretchers

The most common of the commercial stretchers is the rigid-pole, canvas stretcher. It has hinged bracing bars at right angles between the rigid poles at either end that must be locked in the extended position before the stretcher is used.

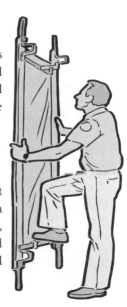

Improvised stretchers

If a commercially prepared stretcher is not available, you can improvise one by using a tabletop, door, or two rigid poles and a blanket, clothing or grain sacks. Don't use non-rigid stretchers like this for casualties with suspected head or spinal injuries.

Principles for stretcher use

Complete all essential first aid and immobilization before moving the casualty onto a stretcher.

2

◆ Bring the blanketed and padded stretcher to the casualty, rather than moving the casualty to the stretcher.

◆ As the first aider in charge, take the position that permits you to watch and control the most sensitive area of the body, usually at the head and shoulders, or the injured part.

◆ Tell the bearers what each is expected to do. If the move is difficult, and time permits, it's a good idea to practise with a simulated casualty. This reduces risks and reassures the conscious casualty.

◆ Use clear commands to ensure smooth, coordinated movements.

Test an improvised stretcher with someone equal to or heavier than the casualty to ensure that it will hold.

Check the clearance of an improvised stretcher to ensure that it will pass through hallways, doors and stairways without harm to the casualty.

Improvised blanket stretcher

1 Place the blanket flat on the ground and place a pole one-third of the way from one end. Fold the one-third length of blanket over the pole.

2 Place the second pole parallel to the first so that it is on the doubled part of the blanket, about 15 cm (6 in) from the doubled edge.

3 Fold the remaining blanket over the two poles. The casualty's weight on the blanket holds the folds in place.

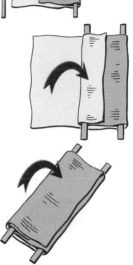

Improvised jacket stretcher

A non-rigid stretcher can also be improvised from two jackets and two or four poles.

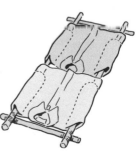

1 Button and zipper the jackets closed and pull the sleeves inside out so that the sleeves are inside. Lay the jackets on the ground so that the top edge of one jacket meets the bottom edge of the other.

2 Pass the poles through the sleeves of the two jackets on either side to complete the stretcher.

3 If the casualty is tall, prepare another jacket as before and add it to the stretcher with the head of the jacket towards the middle.

Four-bearer method—no blanket

1   All bearers kneel on their left knees, three on one side of the casualty and one on the other, as shown below. Bearer 4 helps in lifting and lowering the casualty, and also places the stretcher under the casualty.

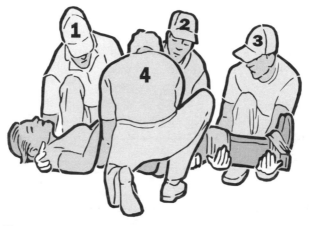

2   Bearer #4 joins hands with bearers 1 and 2. When assured that each bearer has a firm hold on the casualty, bearer 1 directs the others to "Get ready to lift" and then gives the command "Lift." Lift the casualty smoothly to the height of the raised knees.

3   On bearer #1's command "Rest," the casualty is gently laid on the raised knees of bearers 1, 2 and 3. Bearer 1 tells bearer 4 to position the stretcher. Bearer 4 then resumes his position supporting the casualty by linking his hands with one from each of bearers 1 and 2.

4   Position the stretcher.

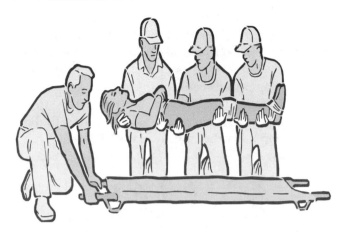

5   When everyone is in position, bearer #1 instructs the team to, "Get ready to lower" and then, "lower." The team lowers the casualty gently onto the stretcher. Secure the casualty to the stretcher.

2

Three-bearer method, no blanket

The three-bearer method is essentially the same as the four-bearer method, except the first aider and one bearer share the weight on one side of the casualty. The third bearer links hands with the first aider from the opposite side to take up the weight of the trunk. The casualty is lifted and rested on the bearers' knees while the stretcher is positioned and bearer 3 links hands again with the first aider to help lower the casualty to the stretcher.

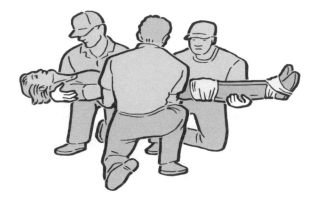

If there are enough bearers to carry the stretcher, walk beside the stretcher to watch the casualty and the route.

Carrying a stretcher

A stretcher may be carried by two or four bearers. As the first aider in charge, decide on the carrying method and give clear instructions to the bearers. After the casualty has been strapped to the stretcher, position yourself so you can watch the casualty and at the same time give direction to the other bearers.

Assign the remaining bearers (depending whether you are two or four) to respective corners or ends of the stretcher. Bearers crouch by the carrying handles of the stretcher, facing in the direction of travel.

◆ When the bearers have a firm footing and a good grip on the stretcher, give the command, "Get ready to lift," and then, "Lift."

◆ Ask the bearers if they are ready. When they are, give the command, "Go forward."

◆ When it is necessary to stop, give the commands "Stop," Get ready to lower," and then, "Lower."

To ensure the smoothest carry for the casualty:

◆ four bearers carrying a stretcher step off together on the foot nearest the stretcher and keep in step

◆ two bearers step off on opposite feet and walk out-of-step

Although stretcher casualties are usually carried feet first, certain conditions call for a head-first carry:

◆ leg injuries during a long downhill carry or when descending stairs, a head-first carry decreases pressure on the lower limbs and minimizes discomfort

◆ uphill carries and going up stairs if there are no

2

injuries to the legs—a head-first carry decreases blood flow to the casualty's head and is more comfortable

◆ loading an ambulance or transferring the casualty to a bed—it is safer to do this head first, and easier to watch the casualty

Obstacles

When crossing uneven ground, a stretcher should be carried by four bearers and kept as level as possible. Bearers must adjust the height of the stretcher to compensate for dips and rises in the terrain.

Crossing a wall

Avoid crossing a wall, even if it means a longer carry. Where a wall must be crossed, follow these steps:

1 Lift the stretcher onto the wall so that the front handles are just over it. The rear bearers hold the stretcher level while the front bearers cross the wall. All lift together and the stretcher is moved forward until the rear handles rest on the wall.

2 The front bearers hold the stretcher level until the rear bearers have crossed the wall and resumed their positions at the rear of the stretcher.

3 The stretcher is then lowered to continue the journey.

Extrication

Extrication is the process of freeing casualties who are trapped or entangled in a vehicle or collapsed structure and cannot free themselves. Provide as much support as possible to the casualty during extrication. Whenever possible, give essential first aid and immobilize the injuries before the casualty is moved.

2

Urgent extrication

When there is an immediate danger and you are alone and must move a casualty from a vehicle, proceed as follows:

1   If necessary, disentangle the person's feet from the vehicle. Ease your forearm under the person's armpit on the exit side, extending your hand to support the chin.

2   Ease the person's head gently backward to rest on your shoulder while keeping the neck as rigid as possible.

3   Ease your other forearm under the armpit on the opposite side and hold the wrist of the casualty's arm which is nearest the exit.

4   Establish a firm footing and swing around with the person, keeping as much rigidity in the neck as possible. Drag the casualty from the vehicle to a safe distance with as little twisting as possible.

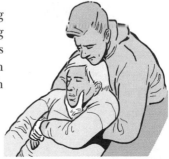

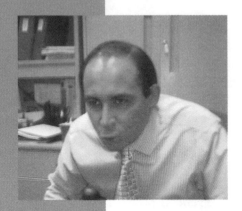

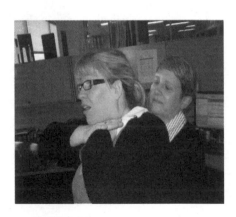

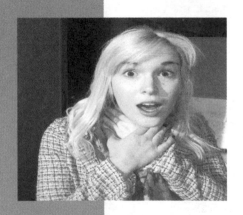

CHAPTER 3

AIRWAY AND BREATHING EMERGENCIES

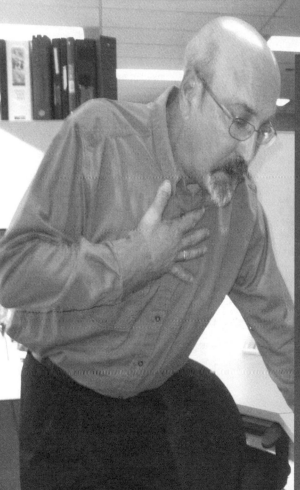

♦ *Effective breathing*

♦ *Ineffective breathing*

♦ *Breathing emergencies caused by injuries*

♦ *First aid for a severe asthma attack*

♦ *First aid for a severe allergic reaction*

♦ *Air exchange*

♦ *Signs of choking*

♦ *First aid for choking*

♦ *How to prevent choking*

Airway and breathing emergencies

3

A clear airway and continuous, effective breathing are vital for life. When a person's breathing is affected through injury or illness, his life can be in immediate danger. As a first aider, you have to be able to recognize a breathing emergency very quickly and know what first aid to give—the casualty's life may depend on it.

Hypoxia

Airway and breathing emergencies cause a lack of oxygen in the blood. This condition, called **hypoxia** can damage vital tissues and eventually cause death if not corrected. The causes of hypoxia are grouped under three headings:

- ◆ **lack of oxygen** —for example:

  - ❖ the oxygen level is low, such as at a high altitude

  - ❖ the oxygen is displaced by other gases, such as a build up of silo gas in a grain silo on a farm or hydrogen sulphide (H2S) in an industrial setting

  - ❖ the oxygen in a small space is used up—for instance where a person is trapped in a confined space and suffocates

- ◆ **blocked airway**—for example:

  - ❖ the casualty chokes on a foreign object, such as food

  - ❖ the unconscious casualty is lying face up and his airway is blocked by the tongue

  - ❖ the casualty's airway becomes swollen due to an allergic reaction

◆ **abnormal heart and lung function**—where the heart and lungs are not working properly due to:

❖ an illness such as chronic obstructive pulmonary disease, pneumonia or congestive heart failure

❖ an injury to the head, spine, chest, etc.

❖ a drug overdose or poisoning

Requirements for effective breathing

To breathe effectively, we need at least the following:

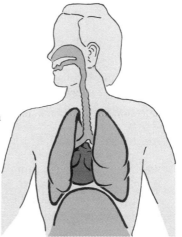

◆ a functioning control centre in the brain and an intact spinal cord so the brain can control breathing

◆ a good supply of oxygen

◆ an open airway

◆ a chest wall that is able to expand and relax

◆ one functioning lung

Signs of normal, effective breathing

The most important signs the first aider uses to assess breathing are rate, rhythm and depth.

Breathing rate is the number of breaths (inhalations and exhalations) in one minute. The normal breathing rate varies for infants, children and adults. The table on the next page gives the range of normal breathing rates for different ages. The table also gives the rates that are too slow and too fast for each age group. A breathing rate that is too slow or too fast is a sign of a breathing emergency.

Breathing rates – breaths per minute

age group	range of normal rates	too slow	too fast
infant (under 1 year)	30 to 50	below 25	above 60
child (1 to 8 years of age)	20 to 30	below 15	above 40
adult(over 8 years of age)	10 to 20	below 10	above 30

3

Breathing **rhythm** refers to the interval between breaths. In normal breathing, the intervals are even and breathing is effortless—this is regular breathing. In irregular breathing, the intervals between breaths are uneven. This usually indicates a respiratory disorder or distress.

Breathing **depth** refers to the amount of air moved in and out of the lungs with each breath. A deep breath draws in more air than a shallow one. Learn to recognize the difference between normal breathing depth, shallow and deep breathing.

Other signs of normal breathing include:

◆ breathing that is quiet and effective

◆ equal expansion of both sides of the chest when the person inhales

◆ the person is alert and relaxed

◆ skin colour is normal

◆ speaking without taking a breath every few words

Signs of ineffective breathing

When a person is breathing effortlessly, we can assume the body is getting the oxygen it needs to function and that breathing is effective. When a person is not getting enough oxygen, the body responds by breathing faster and deeper.

If this increased effort is unable to supply the body's need for oxygen, breathing becomes ineffective. As a first aider, you need to be able to tell the difference between breathing that is somewhat ineffective—where the person's life is not in immediate danger, and breathing that is very ineffective—where the persons's life is in immediate danger. When person has severe difficulty breathing his breathing is ineffective.

3

Look for the signs and symptoms below. Notice whether the person's condition changes over time. If a casualty with breathing difficulty becomes drowsy, we can assume that the brain is not getting enough oxygen. Drowsiness is an indication that the breathing difficulties are severe and medical help is needed urgently.

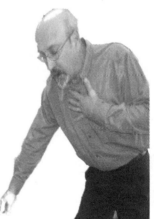

◆ person may be anxious and afraid

◆ breathing is difficult (dyspnea)—
   the casualty is struggling for breath
   or gasping for air

◆ breathing rate may be too fast or
   too slow

◆ breathing rhythm may be irregular

◆ breathing depth may be too shallow
   or too deep

◆ breathing may be noisy or raspy

◆ person may say he's "getting tired" from trying to
   breathe

◆ the person may be sweaty from working so hard at
   breathing

◆ decreased level of consciousness

◆ the lips, ears and fingernail beds turn blue—called cyanosis

◆ chest movement may be abnormal—the chest goes in and the abdomen puffs out during inhalation

◆ there may be little or no chest movement or breathing effort

3

 First aid for ineffective breathing

Ineffective breathing is a life-threatening breathing emergency. Always send or go for medical help at the first sign of a breathing emergency.

Give first aid for ineffective breathing as soon as you see that breathing is ineffective, or when the situation suggests that breathing could become ineffective. The first aid for ineffective breathing has two parts:

1   Give first aid for the injury or condition and if possible, position the casualty to make breathing easier, usually semi-sitting

2   Monitor the casualty's breathing. If breathing stops or becomes ineffective, get medical help immediately. If the casualty loses consciousness and breathing is absent, begin CPR with compressions (see Chapter 4).

The table on the next page lists some of the causes of breathing emergencies. To give first aid, first determine the cause of the breathing emergency, then decide on the best first aid actions.

Causes of airway and breathing emergencies

Injuries	Illnesses	Poisoning
broken ribs	asthma	inhaled poison – e.g. carbon monoxide or H2S poisoning
near drowning	stroke	
knife or gunshot wound	allergic reaction	swallowed poison – e.g. household cleaners or medication overdose
burns to the face or airway	pneumonia	
head injury	congestive heart failure	injected poison – e.g. bee sting
compression of the chest preventing chest expansion	emphysema/bronchitis	

3

Breathing emergencies caused by injuries

If a person is experiencing breathing difficulties following an injury to the body, examine the site of the injury to determine the exact cause. A severe **head injury** could disrupt the nerves controlling breathing and result in ineffective breathing. **Facial injuries** including injuries to the nose and mouth could result in the airway being blocked by loose teeth, dentures, blood or body fluids.

A **chest injury** can damage the rib cage as well as the lungs resulting in severe breathing difficulty. An **open chest injury** results from a penetrating object that breaks through the skin and may cause serious internal damage to the ribs, sternum, lungs, heart or nerves that control breathing. A **closed chest injury** is the result of an impact with a solid object. This can happen in a car crash when the casualty is thrown against the steering wheel or dashboard. The impact may be sufficient to break the ribs and sternum and cause serious damage to internal structures.

If the mechanism of injury suggests a chest injury, and there is difficulty breathing, or if the casualty complains of pain in the chest carefully expose and examine the area. Two serious complications of chest injuries are pneumothorax and flail chest. For more information on these injuries see information on chest injuries on page 188 and 254. In these situations medical help is needed right away.

Inhalation injuries

Inhalation injuries happen when the casualty inhales hot steam or hot (superheated) air, smoke or poisonous chemicals, or carbon monoxide (the most common inhalation injury in a fire).

Inhalation injuries are the most common cause of death from a fire in a building. An inhalation injury is always considered a life-threatening breathing emergency. It can be many hours after inhaling the hot air or poisonous gas that breathing is seriously affected. For this reason, every casualty of an inhalation injury needs to be transported to medical help. Only a medical doctor can determine the extent of the injuries.

Signs and symptoms of inhalation injuries

Signs of hypoxia:

◆ dizziness, restlessness, confusion, unconsciousness

◆ pallor or cyanosis

Signs of severe breathing difficulty:

◆ noisy breathing

◆ abnormal breathing rate or depth

◆ pain during breathing

Signs of being close to heat:

◆ burns on the face, especially the mouth and nose

◆ singed hair on the face or head

Signs of breathing smoke:

◆ sooty or smoky smell on breath

◆ sore throat, hoarseness, barking cough, difficulty
   swallowing

First aid for an inhalation injury

1   Begin ESM—do a scene survey. Make sure you can
       give first aid safely without putting yourself in danger.

2   Do a primary survey. Give first aid for the ABCs. Make
       sure the casualty has a supply of fresh air.

3   Make breathing easier for the casualty—place him
       in the semi-sitting position and loosen tight clothing
       at the neck, chest and waist.

4   Monitor breathing closely. If breathing stops, begin
       CPR starting with compressions.

5   Give ongoing casualty care until handover to
       medical help including first aid for shock.

Breathing emergencies caused by illness

If the person has trouble breathing and there is no reason
to suspect an injury or poisoning, the breathing difficulty
is probably related to an illness. Illnesses that can lead
to severe breathing difficulties include asthma, allergies,
chronic obstructive pulmonary disease (e.g. emphysema),
congestive heart failure and pneumonia. The basic first aid
for all these emergencies is the same.

3

 First aid for breathing emergencies caused by illness

1 Begin ESM.

2 Perform a scene survey and send for medical help if required.

3 Complete a primary survey. If the casualty is experiencing breathing difficulty, place him in the best position for breathing—usually the semi-sitting position.

4 Begin a secondary survey. Find out the history of the incident using **SAMPLE** and assess the vital signs. The history will help you confirm the exact cause of the breathing difficulty.

5 Give appropriate first aid. Ask the casualty if he has any medication for this condition. See page 104 for information on helping with asthma medications, and page 108 for information on medications for severe allergic reactions.

6 Give ongoing casualty care until medical help arrives. Stay with the casualty.

If the casualty becomes unconscious, place him in the recovery position and monitor his breathing closely. If the unconscious casualty stops breathing, begin CPR with compressions (see Chapter 4).

Asthma

Asthma (also called "bronchial asthma") is a respiratory illness in which the person has repeated attacks (asthmatic attacks) of shortness of breath, often with wheezing and coughing. Between attacks, the person has no trouble breathing.

3

Signs and symptoms of a severe asthmatic attack

◆ shortness of breath with obvious trouble breathing

◆ coughing or wheezing (a whistling noise caused by air moving through narrowed airways)—may get louder or stop

◆ fast and shallow breathing

◆ casualty sitting upright trying to breathe

◆ bluish colour in the face (cyanosis)

◆ anxiety, tightness in the chest

◆ fast pulse rate, signs of shock

◆ restlessness at first, and then fatigue—the person becomes tired from trying so hard to breathe

First aid for a severe asthma attack

1   Begin ESM—do a scene survey and a primary survey. As soon as you identify a severe asthma attack, send for medical help.

2   Have the casualty stop any activity and place him in the most comfortable position for breathing. This is usually sitting upright with arms resting on a table.

3   Help the casualty take his prescribed medication.

4   Give ongoing casualty care. Stay with the casualty until medical help takes over. Give plenty of reassurance since fear and anxiety may cause the casualty to breathe faster, making the situation worse.

How to help a casualty take medication for a severe asthmatic attack

A person with asthma may carry medication in the form of a metered-dose **inhaler** (puffer). Usually the person can give himself this medication without help. If the person needs help, a first aider can assist.

An inhaler delivers a premeasured amount of medication. Always read and follow the manufacturer's instructions. Check the prescription label to confirm the casualty's name and expiry date.

Shake the container, then remove the cap.

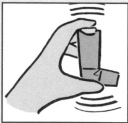

To help a casualty with asthma medication

 Tell the casualty to breathe out completely in a relaxed manner, then to breathe in slowly and deeply—as she does, press the canister to release the medication. The cannister can be in the mouth or approx 4 fingerwidths from the mouth.

 Tell the casualty to hold her breath for 10 seconds so the medication can spread out in the lungs. Then tell her to breathe normally, so the medication won't be expelled. If more doses are needed, wait at least 30-60 seconds before repeating these steps.

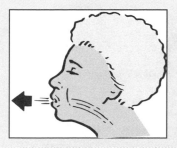

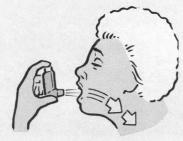

Using a spacer (aero chamber)

When the medication comes out of the inhaler, it may be deposited on the back of the throat. To reduce this problem, use a spacer. It traps the particles of the spray, allowing the casualty to inhale more effectively.

Small children and other casualties who have difficulty coordinating their inhaling with the release of the medication, will find a spacer helpful. It allows them to inhale two or three times before the medication is completely dispelled. A mask can be attached to the device to make taking the medication easier.

If the casualty complains of throat irritation after using the inhaler, have her gargle or rinse her mouth with water.

If the casualty is unable to breathe in deeply before using the inhaler, using the spacer and having the casualty take three or four normal breaths from the spacer will help.

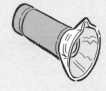

Spacer   Inhaler

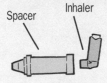

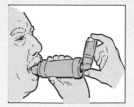

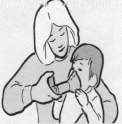

3

Sudden Infant Death Syndrome (SIDS)

There is one breathing emergency that every new parent knows of and dreads—sudden infant death syndrome, or SIDS. Also called crib death, SIDS is the unexplained death of an apparently healthy infant. The infant dies suddenly and unexpectedly, usually while sleeping. One infant per 1,000 die of SIDS in Canada. This makes SIDS the leading cause of death for infants older than four months. SIDS is not likely to occur after one year of age.

First aid for SIDS

The first aid for SIDS is the same as for any unresponsive infant (see page 141). Your actions include:

◆ assess responsiveness

◆ open the airway

◆ assess breathing

◆ if there is no breathing, begin CPR with compressions

◆ get medical help as quickly as possible

Reducing risk factors

Although the exact cause(s) of SIDS is unknown, you can help reduce the risk of SIDS by:*

◆ putting the baby to sleep on his back on a firm, flat surface

◆ keeping the baby in a smoke-free environment

◆ not using bumper pads, quilts, duvets or pillow cases in the crib

◆ not overheating the baby

◆ breast-feeding the baby, if possible

More about SIDS

When a baby dies of SIDS, it is nobody's fault. Although we can reduce the risk factors for SIDS, we cannot prevent it. When even doctors cannot explain the cause, SIDS deaths seem very mysterious and many parents blame themselves or each other. They think it was something they did, or did not do. Sometimes the baby has seen the doctor just before dying, so the parents blame the doctor. But there is no way to tell if a baby is going to die of SIDS. Most babies who have died of SIDS were well fed, well cared for, and seemed to be in good health.

A baby who dies of SIDS does not suffer. The baby does not cry out or struggle in any way. SIDS is not caused by smothering. Occasionally a baby who died of SIDS is found face down and covered in blankets, which may suggest smothering, but this is rarely the case. Most SIDS deaths occur when there is no chance of smothering or strangulation.

For more information on SIDS

Canadian Foundation for the Study of Infant Deaths

60 James St. Suite 403

St. Catharines, ON

L2R 7E7

1-800-END-SIDS

Email: sidsinfo@sidscanada.org

http://www.sidscanada.org

* source: The Canadian Foundation for the Study of Infant Deaths, Canadian Institute for Child Health, Canadian Pediatric Society, and Health Canada

Severe allergic reaction

A life-threatening breathing emergency can result from a severe allergic reaction called **anaphylaxis** (an-a-fi-lak-sis). This reaction usually happens when a substance to which the casualty is very sensitive enters the body. Anaphylaxis can also be caused by exercise or the cause may be unknown. Anaphylaxis is a serious medical emergency that needs urgent medical attention.

Anaphylaxis can happen within seconds, minutes or hours of a substance entering the body. As a rule, the sooner the casualty's body reacts, the worse the reaction will be.

3

 First aid for a severe allergic reaction

1 Begin ESM—do a scene survey and a primary survey. As soon as you identify a severe allergic reaction, send for medical help.

2 Provide first aid. Stop any activity and place the casualty in the most comfortable position for breathing—usually sitting upright.

3 Help the casualty take his prescribed medication. Some people with known allergies carry medication with them. See page 108 for information on helping give the type of medication.

4 Give ongoing casualty care. Stay with the casualty until medical help takes over. Give plenty of reassurance. Fear and anxiety will make the casualty's condition worse.

How to help with medication for anaphylaxis

Anaphylaxis medication (epinephrine) is injected into the body with a needle. The two products available in North America are explained here. These devices are designed for simple use and give the right amount of medication with each injection. If the casualty cannot give the injection to himself, you may have to assist the casualty with the medication.

3

EpiPen® or Twinject® Auto-injector

Both auto-injectors are disposable drug-delivery systems with a spring-activated, concealed needle.

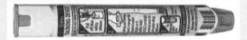

An **EpiPen®** Auto-injector delivers a single dose of medication. A casualty may have more than one auto-injector for multiple doses.

Check the expiry date

LOT 1A2345
EXP DEC 96

The **Twinject®** Auto-injector delivers two doses of medication in a single device. (The second dose is delivered by a manual injection).

In both cases, it is important to be familiar with, and follow the manufacturer's instructions.

To use the auto-injector

1

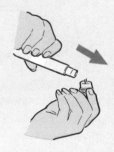

Remove the EpiPen® from the storage tube.

Hold it firmly with the orange tip downward.

Remove the blue safety release.

Remove the TwinJect® from the storage tube.

Remove green cap marked 1 to reveal a red tip. Never touch the red tip.

Pull off the green end cap marked 2.

Only use the auto-injector on the fleshy part of the mid-outer thigh.

Auto-injectors can be given through lightweight clothing.

Press the orange tip of the EpiPen® or red tip of the Twinject®, firmly into the mid-outer thigh until the unit activates. Hold the auto-injector in place for several seconds, then pull it straight out.

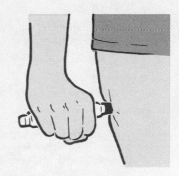

After the injection, keep the casualty warm and avoid any exertion.

Call 9-1-1 as soon as you have given the first dose and describe the casualty's signs and symptoms. Tell the dispatcher that one dose of the auto-injector has been given. If a second dose is available it is recommended you seek medical advice regarding another dose.

This will require a second EpiPen® or the administration of the second dose of the Twinject® which is delivered by manual injection.

Individuals who are feeling faint or dizzy because of impending shock should be placed flat on their back unless they are vomiting or experiencing respiratory distress. It is important that the casualty does not sit or stand immediately as this could cause a drop in blood pressure.

The medication will begin to wear off within 10 to 20 minutes—get medical help right away.

◆ Check the expiry date. If the only auto-injector available is an expired product, it may still be life-saving and should be administered if indicated if the liquid remains clear

◆ If you or anyone else is injected by mistake, get medical help.

What to do with the auto-injector

Follow manufacturer's directions for proper care of the used device. Put the used unit back in the storage tube and take it to the hospital with the casualty.

For more information on the **EpiPen®** Auto-injector check out www.epipen.ca

For more information on the **Twinject®** Auto-injector check out www.twinject.ca

Hyperventilation

Hyperventilation is a condition of "overbreathing." It can be caused by acute anxiety or emotional stress, drug withdrawal, poisoning, or for no obvious reason. A hyperventilation attack can be very dramatic—the casualty may be very frightened, and the people with the casualty may also become upset.

3

Signs and symptoms of hyperventilation

◆ breathing is fast and deep

◆ the casualty may say: "I can feel my heart pounding!"

◆ "I feel like I am smothering and can't get enough air!"

◆ "I'm having trouble swallowing."

◆ pulse is rapid, skin colour is usually good

◆ headache, chest pains, dizziness, tingling, shaking.

First aid for hyperventilation

The aim of first aid for hyperventilation is to calm the person and reassure him. In stress-related hyperventilation, quietly reassure and encourage the casualty to slow the rate of respiration ease the symptoms. Ask the casualty to match your normal rate and depth of breathing.

The casualty who is hyperventilating should be taken to medical help for evaluation and further care. Some serious medical conditions look like hyperventilation.

Choking

A person chokes when the airway is partly or completely blocked and airflow to the lungs is reduced or cut off. The choking casualty either has trouble breathing or cannot breathe at all. A choking casualty may die if first aid for choking is not given right away.

open and clear airway

partly blocked airway

partial blockage

Air exchange – good, poor or none

A person's airway can be either partly or completely blocked. With a partially blocked airway, there is either **good air exchange or poor air exchange**. With good air exchange, the obstruction is mild and person can still cough forcefully, breathe and speak. With poor air exchange, the obstruction is severe and the person cannot cough forcefully, has trouble breathing, or cannot speak. With a completely

completely blocked airway

foreign object

Causes of choking

Foreign Objects	The Tongue	Swelling
◆ in infants and children—food, toys, buttons, coins, etc.	◆ tongue falls to the back of the throat when lying on back	◆ injury to the throat area causes swelling of the airway
		◆ illness causes swelling, e.g. allergic reaction, asthma, epiglottitis, croup

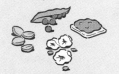

◆ in adults—gulping drinks with food in your mouth

◆ in elderly people— food, pills

◆ saliva, blood or vomit pools in the throat

swollen airway

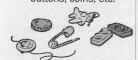

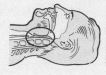

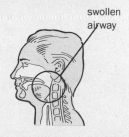

blocked airway, there is no air exchange—coughing, breathing and speaking are impossible.

What happens when a person chokes

Choking is a life-threatening emergency. When the air supply to the lungs is cut off, the person's face immediately becomes red or "flushed". Shortly after, as the oxygen in the body is used up, the face becomes grey and the lips and ear lobes become blue. This change in colour is called cyanosis. Soon, the person becomes unconscious and eventually the heart stops beating.

Signs of choking

The most obvious sign of choking is grabbing the throat. You need to know how to recognize whether a choking person has a mild or severe obstruction because the first aid is different for each.

Mild obstruction

- able to speak

- signs of distress—eyes show fear

- forceful coughing

- wheezing and gagging between coughs

- red or "flushed" face

- grabbing the throat

Severe obstruction

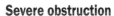

- not able to speak

- signs of distress— eyes show fear

- weak or no coughing

- high-pitched noise or no noise when trying to breathe

- grey face and blue lips and ears

- grabbing the throat

First aid for choking

There are two choking situations you may have to deal with:

◆ a conscious choking person who may become unconscious while you are giving first aid

◆ an unconscious person who, you discover through your first aid actions, has a blocked airway

3

The first aid you give depends on the casualty's age. Ages are guidelines only; the casualty's size must be also considered. There are variations in the techniques for a casualty who is pregnant, much larger than the rescuer or in a wheelchair.

First aid for a choking adult

1 Begin ESM—do a scene survey

2 If the casualty can cough forcefully, speak or breathe, don't touch her. Tell her to try to cough up the object. If a mild obstruction lasts for a few minutes, get medical help.

If you think there might be a severe obstruction, check by asking, "Are you choking?" If the casualty cannot cough forcefully, speak or breathe, use back blows followed by abdominal thrusts to remove the blockage.

3 To give back blows and abdominal thrusts;

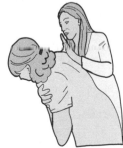

◆ support the casualty's upper body and help her lean forward. Give up to five sharp blows between the shoulder blades using the heel of your hand.

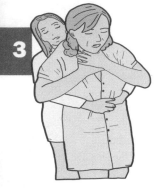

3

◆ If the obstruction is not cleared, begin abdominal thrusts. Stand behind the casualty ready to support her if she becomes unconscious.

◆ Place a foot between the casualty's feet for a solid position

◆ Place your fist midline, just above the belly button

◆ Hold the fist with the other hand and pull inward/upward giving 5 sharp and forceful thrusts

◆ Give each abdominal thrust with the intention of removing the object. Use only your fist— make sure you don't press against the ribs with your forearms.

4   If the object is not removed, repeat back blows and abdominal thrusts until either the object is removed or the casualty becomes unconscious. If the airway is cleared, give ongoing casualty care as described on page 124.

If the casualty becomes unconscious, don't panic. Lower her to the ground. Send someone to call for medical help and get an AED if available.

If choking is caused by swelling of the airway from an infection, injury or allergic reaction, back blows and abdominal thrusts won't work–get medical help quickly.

Begin compressions immediately. After the first 30 compressions, check the mouth. Remove the foreign object if you can see it. Try to give 2 breaths and continue to give CPR as described in Chapter 4. Check the mouth before each attempt to ventilate, until ventilations are successful.

First aid for a choking casualty much larger than the rescuer

If a choking casualty is very large compared to the rescuer, or if the casualty is in the late stages of pregnancy, abdominal thrusts may not be effective. Instead of abdominal thrusts, use chest thrusts as described below along with the back blows described on page 113.

3

Chest thrusts for a conscious choking casualty

1   Stand behind the casualty and wrap your arms around her chest.

2   Keep your arms horizontal and snug up under her armpits.

3   Place your fist against the lower half of the breastbone with the thumb-side in.

4   Hold your fist with your other hand. Pull inward forcefully. Give each thrust with the intention of removing the blockage.

5   Give 5 back blows and 5 chest thrusts until either the object is removed or the casualty becomes unconscious.

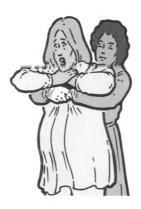

Choking adult – self-help

If you begin to choke on an object, what should you do?

1   Don't panic, though that's not easy. If there are people around, get their attention—grab your throat to show them you are choking—this is the universal sign of choking. **Do not isolate yourself from others**.

2   If you can cough forcefully, try to cough up the object.

3   If you can't cough forcefully, breathe or speak, and there is no one else to help, you can help yourself as shown below. Use either your hands, a piece of furniture or whatever gives the best effect.

Put a fist, thumb-side in, midline on your abdomen just above your hips.

Hold the fist with your other hand and pull inward/ upward forcefully.

Give yourself abdominal thrusts until you can cough forcefully, breathe or speak.

If you are very large or in the late stages of pregnancy, give yourself chest thrusts instead. Place a fist, thumb-side down, in the middle of your chest. With your head turned to the side, fall against a wall hard enough to produce a chest thrust.

A second method is to use a solid object like the back of a chair, a table or the edge of a counter.

◆ Position yourself so the object is just above your hips.

◆ Press forcefully and quickly to produce an abdominal thrust—keep giving yourself thrusts until you can cough forcefully, breathe or speak.

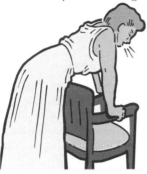

If you are alone and choking, you must get help quickly— you will become unconscious within minutes.

Do whatever is necessary to get someone's attention. If you have 9-1-1 emergency service in your area, call for help. In some areas, the 9-1-1 operator can see on the equipment the address of the phone the caller is using and help will be sent even though you cannot tell them what's wrong.

How abdominal thrusts work

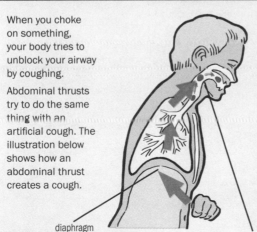

When you choke on something, your body tries to unblock your airway by coughing.

Abdominal thrusts try to do the same thing with an artificial cough. The illustration below shows how an abdominal thrust creates a cough.

An abdominal thrust pushes the diaphragm up towards the lungs very quickly. This forces the air from the lungs up the airway and hopefully blows the obstruction out.

For the best effect, the fist has to be in the correct place. Keep your forearms off the abdomen and make each thrust a strong and sudden movement.

diaphragm

foreign object

First aid for a choking casualty in a wheelchair

The way you do abdominal thrusts for someone in a wheelchair depends largely on the type of wheelchair. If you can reach around from behind the wheelchair, give abdominal thrusts and back blows as you would for any conscious casualty of the same age. If you cannot reach around the wheelchair, use the technique shown below.

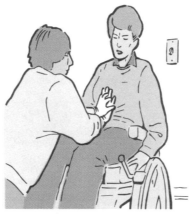

◆ position the wheelchair against a wall

◆ put the wheelchair brake on

◆ put the heel of one hand, with the other on top, in the middle of the abdomen, well below the notch where the ribs meet

◆ give sudden, inward/upward thrusts until the object is removed or the casualty becomes unconscious

If a doctor, physiotherapist or other health professional has shown you a different way of giving abdominal thrusts to a person in your care, use the method that you prefer.

If the casualty becomes unconscious, take her out of the wheelchair.

◆ grip the casualty's clothing

◆ lower yourself and the casualty to the ground using the strength in your legs and not your back as much as possible

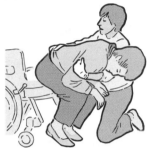

◆ pull the casualty forward supporting her with your arm and leg

◆ supporting the casualty, and protecting the head as

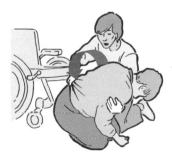

much as possible, roll the casualty to the floor to a face-up position

Send someone to call for medical help and get an AED if available. Begin compressions immediately. After the first 30 compressions, check the mouth. Remove the foreign object if you can see it. Give 2 breaths and give CPR as described in Chapter 4. Check the mouth before each attempt to ventilate until the airway is clear.

3

 First aid for a choking child

First aid for a choking child involves the same steps as for an adult. It is important to take into account the difference in size between youself and the casualty.

1   Begin ESM—do a scene survey. Identify yourself as a first aider to the parent or guardian and offer to help. If no parent or guardian is present, implied consent is assumed.

2   Find out how badly the child is choking. Ask, "Are you choking?"

   If the child can speak, breathe or cough, don't touch him. Tell her to try to cough up the object. If this partial blockage lasts for more than a few minutes, get medical help.

3   Support the child's upper body and help her lean forward. Give up to five sharp blows between the shoulder blades using the heel of your hand.

4   If back blows are not successful, kneel behind the casualty so you are at the correct height to give abdominal thrusts. Position your hands as you did for the adult and give five sharp thrusts.

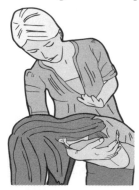

Continue to give a combination of back blows and abdominal thrusts until the airway is cleared or the child becomes unconscious.

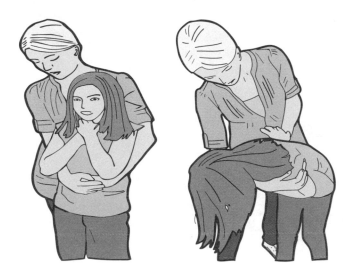

If the object is removed, give ongoing casualty care as described on page 124.

5   If the child becomes unconscious, don't panic. Lower her to the ground. Send someone to call for medical help and get an AED if available. Begin compressions immediately. After the first 30 compressions, check the mouth. Remove the foreign object if you can see it. Give 2 breaths and give CPR as described in Chapter 4. Check the mouth before each attempt to ventilate until the airway is clear.

If choking is caused by swelling of the airway from an infection, injury or allergic reaction, back blows and abdominal thrusts won't work–get medical help quickly.

3

Infant choking casualty

Suspect an infant is choking when she suddenly has trouble breathing, even if you haven't seen the baby actually put something into her mouth. Coughing, gagging, and high-pitched, noisy breathing all indicate breathing difficulty. Whenever you suspect an infant is choking, start first aid right away.

 First aid for a choking infant

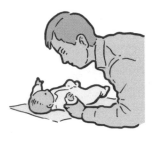

1   Begin ESM—do the scene survey. Identify yourself as a first aider to the parent or guardian and offer to help. If no parent or guardian is present, implied consent is assumed.

2   Assess the baby's breathing. If the baby can cough forcefully or breathe, stand by and don't interfere, let the baby try to cough up the object. If a partial blockage lasts for more than a few minutes, get medical help.

If the baby cannot cough forcefully, cannot breathe, makes a high-pitched noise when trying to breathe or starts to turn blue, give back blows and chest thrusts to try to relieve the blockage.

3   Pick the baby up and turn her over. Support the head and neck throughout the movement.

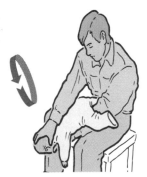

4   Secure the baby between your forearms and turn her face down.

With the baby's head lower than the body, use the heel of your hand to give five forceful back blows between the shoulder blades.

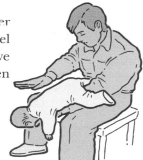

3

5   Turn the baby face up and bring her close to you. Give chest thrusts to create an artificial cough. Give five chest thrusts, each with the intention of removing the object. Use two fingers positioned just below the nipple line.

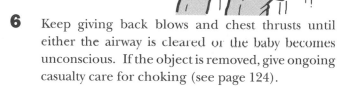

6   Keep giving back blows and chest thrusts until either the airway is cleared or the baby becomes unconscious. If the object is removed, give ongoing casualty care for choking (see page 124).

7   If the baby becomes unconscious, go or send a bystander to call for medical help. Begin CPR with compressions (see Chapter 4). After each set of compressions, check the mouth. If you see the foreign object, remove it. Try to give two breaths and continue CPR checking the mouth each time.

Ongoing casualty care for choking

Your job as a first aider is not over when the airway blockage is removed. When a choking casualty's airway has been cleared, she may be conscious, semi-conscious or unconscious. Continue giving first aid as described below.

If the casualty is conscious

◆ monitor breathing often. Breathing difficulties can develop following a choking incident

◆ stay with the casualty until normal breathing returns

Urge the casualty to see a medical doctor—abdominal thrusts can cause internal injuries

If the casualty is semi-conscious or unconscious

◆ call for medical help if not called already

◆ if the casualty is breathing, place her in the recovery position and give first aid for shock

◆ monitor ABCs closely

◆ stay with the casualty until medical help takes over

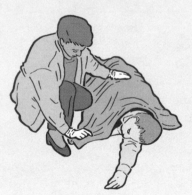

Place a semi-conscious or unconscious casualty into the recovery position.

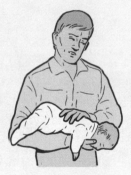

Infant recovery position

3

How to prevent choking

The prevention tips below are based on the most common causes of choking. Use these tips to reduce the risk of choking.

3

Preventing choking in adults

◆ Cut food into small pieces or take small bites when not using a knife and fork

◆ Drink alcohol in moderation. Alcohol causes you to lose the coordination of the muscles used in swallowing, and makes it easier to choke

◆ Don't talk, laugh or gulp drinks with food in your mouth

Preventing choking in children

◆ Supervise children when they are eating.

◆ Don't feed the following food items to children under four years of age:

- nuts   - popcorn
- round candies   - grapes
- hot dogs   - thickly-spread peanut butter

◆ Cut hot dogs in half lengthwise for older children.

◆ Teach children not to run or move about when eating.

◆ Balloons are a common cause of choking—always supervise children when they're playing with balloons.

◆ Check your house regularly for items that could cause choking, especialy under furniture and between the cushions on couches and chairs—coins are a common hazard.

Preventing choking in infants

◆ Inspect all toys for small parts that may come off—keep these toys away from infants.

◆ Only give infants small bite-sized pieces of food, especially when the infant has few teeth or is just learning to eat solids.

◆ Keep all toys out of the baby's crib.

◆ Check pacifiers for small parts or worn nipples. Throw these away immediately.

◆ Don't let infants play with balloons.

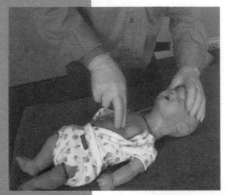

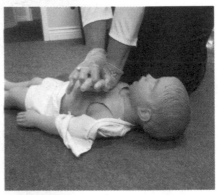

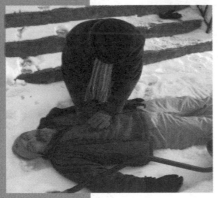

Cardiovascular Emergencies and CPR

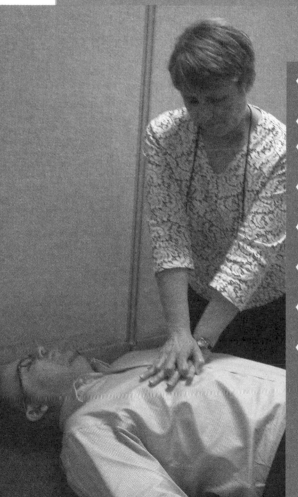

- *Cardiovascular emergencies*

- *Cardiac arrest*

- *First aid for angina/heart attack*

- *First aid for heart failure*

- *First aid for stroke/ TIA*

- *Cardiopulmonary resuscitation (CPR)*

- *Automated external defibrillation (AED)*

- *How to take over CPR from another rescuer*

Introduction

Cardiovascular disease kills more Canadians than any other cause of death. Some of these deaths could be prevented if appropriate first aid were given. Even more of these deaths could be prevented if individuals adopted a heart-healthy lifestyle that reduces the risk of cardiovascular disease. This chapter describes:

4

◆ cardiovascular disease

◆ how to reduce your risk of cardiovascular disease

◆ first aid for cardiovascular emergencies, including

❖ first aid for stroke/TIA

❖ first aid for angina/heart attack

❖ first aid for cardiac arrest, which is CPR

Cardiovascular emergencies

Cardiovascular disease refers to disorders of the heart and blood vessels. High blood pressure and atherosclerosis are cardiovascular disorders. Over time, they can lead to cardiovascular emergencies such as angina, heart attack, congestive heart failure, transient ischemic attack, stroke and cardiac arrest. Each of these is described in this chapter along with the first aid procedures.

High blood pressure

Blood pressure is the pressure of the blood against the inside walls of the blood vessels. Blood pressure goes up and down naturally. When a person is excited or emotionally stressed, blood pressure goes up, but it usually comes down once the excitement has passed. In some people, their blood pressure stays high all the time. This condition of constant high blood pressure is called hypertension. Over time, hypertension damages the tissues of the cardiovascular system. The walls of the blood vessels become thick and lose their elasticity and the heart becomes enlarged.

The changes caused by high blood pressure increase the risk of stroke, heart attack, kidney or eye problems. Unfortunately, hypertension does not always give warning signals—you may feel perfectly well but still have high blood pressure. This is why it is called the silent killer.

4

Narrowing of the arteries

Arteries are the blood vessels that carry blood away from the heart. They become diseased when fatty deposits build up inside them, making the passage for blood narrower. This process of fat deposition and narrowing of the arteries is called atherosclerosis. In the coronary arteries, which carry oxygenated blood to the heart, it is called coronary artery disease.

As an artery gets narrower, less and less blood gets through. When the artery gets too narrow, the tissues on the other side of the narrowing don't get enough oxygenated blood to function normally. Although the signs and symptoms of hardening of the arteries usually don't appear until middle age or later, atherosclerosis often begins in childhood.

Angina

If one of the coronary arteries becomes narrowed or hardened, the blood supply feeding that part of the heart muscle becomes limited. When the heart works harder and needs more blood (e.g. when you run for a bus or shovel snow), it can't get the oxygenated blood it needs through the narrowed coronary artery. This causes pain or discomfort in the chest which may spread to the neck, jaw, shoulders and arms. This pain is called angina pectoris (or "angina"). Angina pain doesn't usually last long, and goes away if the person rests and takes prescribed medication. Many people with angina live normally by taking medication that increases blood flow to the heart.

Heart attack

4

A heart attack happens when heart muscle tissue dies because its supply of oxygenated blood has been cut off. Usually, a blood clot gets stuck in a coronary artery that has been narrowed through atherosclerosis. The supply of blood is cut off and the heart tissue beyond the clot is starved of oxygen. A heart attack can feel just like angina, except the pain doesn't go away with rest and medication. If the heart attack damages the heart's electrical system, or if a lot of the heart muscle is affected, the heart may stop beating properly. This is **cardiac arrest.**

Doctors now have drugs to dissolve a blood clot, but they work best if given right away. This is why you have to call 9-1-1 and get a casualty with a suspected heart attack to the hospital right away—the longer medical help is delayed, the more likely the heart will be damaged or stop beating. The medical term for a heart attack is **myocardial infarction** (my-o-car-dee-al in-fark-shun).

Chain of Survival ™

The Chain of Survival ™

CPR is often what comes to mind when people think of first aid for a heart attack or cardiac arrest. But CPR is only part of the picture. There are 5 links that provide direction to first aiders when helping someone with heart problems.

◆ 1. immediate recognition of a cardiovascular emergency and activation of the community emergency medical services (EMS) system.
This means calling for help . . .quickly

◆ 2. early CPR with an emphasis on chest compressions

◆ 3. rapid defibrillation if required (defibrillation is an electrical shock given to a quivering heart to make it beat properly again)

◆ 4. effective advanced life support

◆ 5. intergrated post-cardiac arrest care

Each of the steps is as important as the others. None of them alone will give the casualty the best chance for survival. Time is a vital ingredient. To give a casualty in cardiac arrest a reasonable chance of survival, CPR must be started immediately followed by defibrillation as quickly as possible. For both procedures, the sooner they happen, the better.

You, the first trained person on the scene, are responsible for initiating the sequence. You must recognize the cardiovascular emergency, call for medical help, start CPR if needed, and apply a defibrillator if trained. You are the crucial first three links in the chain of survival.

Early recognition and denial

The first step is recognizing a cardiovascular emergency. This may be the toughest job you have to do. It's not easy to accept that someone is having a heart attack and could die very soon. This is especially true if the person is a family member or a close friend (family members and friends are often present during a heart attack). The person could still be talking to you and not look as if he is about to die. And perhaps the person is denying anything serious is happening, which often occurs.

On average, casualties take 4½ hours to get to a hospital from the time they first start feeling poorly. One reason for this is that it takes a long time to accept that something serious could be wrong.

It is this wasted time that prevents many lives from being saved. When someone complains of chest pain, you should consider it a serious problem—that's early recognition. The first thing you should do is call for medical help—that's early access

By getting the casualty to the hospital quickly, you will have given her the best chance for survival. If there is no serious problem, you will still have done the right thing and the casualty will have had a complete check-up. On the other hand, if there is a serious problem, you may have saved a life.

Signs and symptoms of angina and a heart attack

◆ the pain may feel like:
  - heaviness in chest
  - tightness in chest
  - squeezing of chest
  - pressure on chest
  - crushing of chest
  - indigestion
  - aching jaw
  - sore arms

◆ other signs and symptoms include:
  - denial
  - fear
  - pale skin
  - nausea, vomiting
  - sweating
  - shortness of breath
  - fatigue
  - shock
  - unconsciousness
  - cardiac arrest

4

 ## First aid for angina/heart attack

A first aider may understand the difference between angina and a heart attack, but a first aider cannot decide whether a casualty is having angina pain or a heart attack—only a medical doctor can do this. For this reason, the first aid for angina and heart attack is the same.

1 Begin ESM—do the scene survey.

2 Do a primary survey. Ask the casualty questions to determine the history.

"Can you show me where it hurts?"

"Have you had this pain before?"

"Do you have medication for this pain?"

3 As soon as you recognize the signs and symptoms of angina/heart attack, call, or have a bystander call, for medical help. If you have to leave to call, place the casualty at rest before you go.

4   Place the casualty at rest to reduce the work the heart has to do. The most comfortable position for the casualty is best. In most cases, the semi-sitting position will be best but this is not always the case. Let the casualty try what has helped before, but don't delay calling medical help while trying different positions to ease the pain.

5   Make the casualty comfortable—loosen tight clothing at the neck, chest and waist. Reassure the casualty to lessen fear and worry—these cause the heart to work harder.

6   Help the conscious casualty to take his prescribed medication. Follow the guidelines below. If the casualty has no prescribed medication or there is no relief after the first dose of the prescribed medication, ask the casualty if he has any allergies to ASA or if a doctor has ever told him not to take ASA. If not, suggest he chew 1 regular ASA tablet or two low dose ASA tablets.

7   If the casualty loses consciousness and stops breathing, start CPR with compressions.

Research has shown that the early administration of ASA can reduce the effects of a heart attack by as much as 20%.

4

Helping with cardiac medication

Only assist a casualty with medication if he is conscious and specifically asks for your help.

Nitroglycerin tablets or sprays are common medications for relief of angina pain. Ask the casualty if he uses drugs to treat erectile dysfunction such as Viagra®. If the person has taken any of these drugs it is recommended they not take nitroglycerin as this may cause a significant decrease in the person's blood pressure. Ensure the medication is prescribed for this person.

Spray under the tongue or place the tablets under the tongue—they aren't to be swallowed. Nitroglycerin may be repeated, if needed, every 5-10 minutes to relieve pain, or until a maximum of three doses have been taken.

4

Congestive heart failure

Heart failure means the heart can't pump blood effectively any more. Chronic heart disease or a previous heart attack may have led to this condition. Since the heart cannot pump properly, blood begins to back up in the lungs, causing breathing problems. The blood also backs up in the rest of the body and causes swelling, as in the ankles.

Signs and symptoms of heart failure

◆ inappropriate shortness of breath, especially when exercising

◆ difficulty breathing when lying flat

◆ blueness around the lips, fingernail beds, ears and other parts of the body

◆ swelling of the ankles

◆ coughing up frothy, pink fluid

 First aid for heart failure

1   Begin ESM—do the scene survey.

2   Do a primary survey. Send or go for medical help and an AED if available.

3   Place the casualty at rest in a semi-sitting position and loosen tight clothing.

4   Reassure the casualty and monitor breathing closely. Be prepared to begin CPR if breathing stops (see page 138).

Stroke

If a blood clot blocks a narrowed artery in the brain and the part of the brain beyond the clot doesn't get the oxygen it needs, the brain tissue dies. This is called a stroke or cerebrovascular accident (CVA). A severe stroke can cause death. A less severe stroke may cause brain damage, which impairs certain body functions, depending on the part of the brain affected. In both heart attack and stroke, hardening of the arteries is the main cause. Over time, the arteries become narrowed and finally a clot blocks a narrowed artery. The difference between the heart attack and the stroke is the final resting place of the clot. A stroke can also be caused by a ruptured artery.

A condition similar to a stroke is a transient ischemic attack (TIA). A TIA is caused by a lack of oxygen to part of the brain. It has the same signs and symptoms as a stroke. A TIA usually lasts from a few minutes to several hours and leaves no permanent brain damage. Although a TIA by itself is not life-threatening, it is a warning sign that a stroke may follow. A TIA that lasts longer than 12 hours is usually considered a stroke. Advise anyone who has a TIA to get medical help.

Signs and symptoms of a stroke/TIA

The signs and symptoms of a stroke/TIA depend on what part of the brain is affected. Often, only one side of the body shows signs because only one side of the brain is affected. Remember F.A.S.T. as a way to check for the signs of a stroke and to get immediate help.

◆ Facial droop—one side of the face doesn't move as well as the other side

◆ Arm drift—have the casualty hold both arms out. One arm may not move or drifts down compared to the other arm

◆ Speech—the casualty slurs words, uses the incorrect words or is not able to speak

◆ Time—get immediate medical help; the earlier a stroke is treated the better the outcome

 First aid for stroke/TIA

A first aider can't tell whether the casualty is having a stroke or a TIA, so the first aid is the same for both. If the signs and symptoms pass after a short while, suggesting the problem was a TIA, advise the casualty to see a doctor. A stroke could soon follow.

1 Begin ESM—do the scene survey. If the casualty is unresponsive, send or go for medical help and an AED if available.

2 Do a primary survey.

3 Place the casualty at rest in the most comfortable position—usually semi-sitting.

4 Give nothing by mouth. If the casualty is thirsty, moisten the lips with a wet cloth.

5 Protect the casualty from injury when he is lifted, moved or during convulsions.

6 Reassure the casualty and keep him warm.

7 If the casualty becomes semiconscious or unconscious, place him in the recovery position. If there is paralysis, position the casualty with the paralyzed side up. This will reduce the chance of tissue or nerve damage to the affected side.

8 Be prepared to begin CPR if breathing stops (see page 138).

Cardiac arrest

When the heart stops pumping, it is in cardiac arrest. Cardiac arrest can happen suddenly or may follow a period of stopped or ineffective breathing, after much of the oxygen in the body is used up. A heart attack causes cardiac arrest when so much heart tissue is damaged that it can't pump blood anymore. Other reasons for cardiac arrest include severe injuries, electrical shock, drug overdose, drowning, suffocation and stroke. When a person's heart has stopped, he is considered clinically dead even though he may still be resuscitated. The first aid for cardiac arrest is cardiopulmonary resuscitation (CPR) as described in the sequence below.

Cardiopulmonary Resuscitation (CPR)

CPR is two basic life support skills put together—artificial respiration and artificial circulation. Artificial respiration provides oxygen to the lungs. Artificial circulation causes blood to flow through the body, but only enough to give a person a chance for survival. The purpose of CPR is to circulate oxygenated blood to the brain and other organs until either the heart starts beating, or medical help takes over.

The CPR sequence follows from the scene survey and primary survey outlined in Chapter 2. When you find an unresponsive casualty, send for help immediately. Then, start the primary survey. If there is no breathing, begin CPR. If an AED (automated external defibrillator) is available, use it as soon as possible. Variations in the CPR sequence are described for situations involving an adult casualty, a child casualty and an infant casualty.

CPR – Adult casualty

1   Begin ESM—start the scene survey.

2   Assess responsiveness. If there is no response, go to step 3.

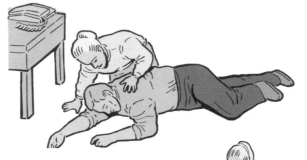

3   Send or go for medical help and an AED if available. Do a primary survey. Open the airway. Check for breathing for at least 5 and no more than 10 seconds.

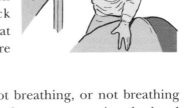

4   If the casualty is not breathing, or not breathing normally, place him face up, protecting the head and neck during any movement.

5   Make sure he is on a firm, flat surface.

Kneel so your hands can be placed mid-chest. Position your hands in the centre of the upper chest and your shoulders directly over your hands. Keep your elbows locked.

6   Give 30 compressions—Push hard—Push Fast! Depress and release the chest rhythmically. Press the heels of the hands straight down on the breastbone. The depth of each compression should be at least 5 cm (2 inches). The pressure and release phases take the same time.

Release pressure and completely remove your weight at the top of each compression to allow chest to return to the resting position.

4

Give compressions at a rate of at least 100 per minute. Count compressions out loud to keep track of how many you have given, and to help keep a steady rhythm.

7 Open the airway by tilting the head and lifting the chin.

8 Breathe into the casualty twice. For an adult casualty, each breath should take about for 1 second. Use enough air to make the chest rise.

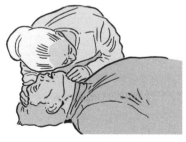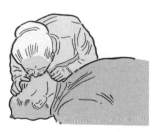

This is one cycle of 30:2 (30 compressions to 2 ventilations).

9 Continue CPR until either an AED is applied, the casualty begins to respond, another first aider or medical help takes over or you are too exhausted to continue.

CPR – Child casualty

1   Begin ESM—start the scene survey. Identify yourself as a first aider to the parent or guardian and offer to help. If no parent or guardian is present, implied consent is assumed.

2   Assess responsiveness. If there is no response ... send a bystander for medical help and an AED if available. If you are alone, give 5 cycles of CPR (approx. 2 minutes) before you go for help. Carry the child with you if possible after the 2 minutes of CPR.

3   Open the airway. Check for breathing for at least 5 and no more than 10 seconds. If the child is not breathing, or not breathing normally, position the child face up and begin CPR with compressions.

4   Make sure the child is on a firm, flat surface and position your hand(s) on the chest for chest compressions.

You may use one or two hands depending on the size of the child.

5   Follow the same steps used for the adult casualty continuing cycles of 30 compressions followed by 2 ventilations. Give compressions at a rate of at least 100 per minute. Depress the chest 1/3 the depth of the chest or about 2 inches (5 cm).

6   Continue CPR until either an AED is applied, the casualty begins to respond, another first aider or medical help takes over or you are too exhausted to continue.

CPR – infant casualty

1 Begin ESM—start the scene survey. Identify yourself as a first aider to the parent or guardian and offer to help. If no parent or guardian is present, implied consent is assumed.

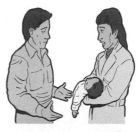

2 Assess responsiveness. Gently tap the baby's feet.

If there is no response, go to step 3.

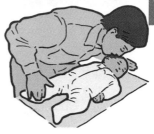

3 Send a bystander for medical help. If you are alone, give 5 cycles of CPR (approx. 2 minutes) before calling for help. Carry the infant with you, if possible, to the telephone.

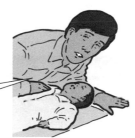

Get medical help. Call an ambulance and tell them an infant is unconscious.

4 Open the airway. Place your ear near the baby's mouth and nose. Check for breathing for at least 5 and up to 10 seconds. If the baby is not breathing, or not breathing normally, place the baby face up and begin CPR.

5   Make sure she is on a firm, flat surface and position your fingers on the chest for chest compressions.

Begin CPR with thirty compressions. Place two fingers on the breastbone just below the nipple line. Push down on the breastbone 1/3 the depth of the chest (1 1/2 inches or about 4 cm).

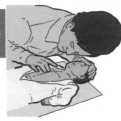

Release the pressure completely but keep your fingers in light contact with the chest. Repeat the pressure and release phases rhythmically so that each phase takes the same amount of time.

Give compressions at a rate of at least 100 per minute.

6   Open the airway by tilting the head and lifting the chin.

Seal your mouth around the baby's mouth and nose and blow in. Move your mouth away and allow the air to escape.

Breathe into the baby twice. Blow for 1 second each time using just enough air to make the chest rise.

CPR for the infant casualty

The back of an infant's head is quite large compared to the rest of her body. This causes the baby's head to come forward and close off her airway.

When giving CPR, it may be helpful to put a thin pad under the shoulders to help keep the airway open—but don't waste time looking for a pad.

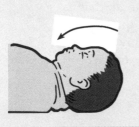

An infant's head flexes forward when she's lying on her back

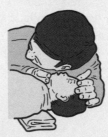

A thin pad under the shoulders helps keep the airway open

7 Continue CPR at a ratio of 30:2 (thirty compressions to two ventilations) until either the casualty starts to respond, another first aider or medical help takes over or you are too exhausted to continue.

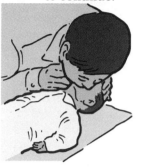 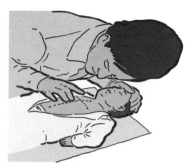

Compression only CPR

CPR guidelines stress early recognition of the emergency and stress the importance of calling 9-1-1 or the local emergency number if you find someone collapsed and unresponsive.

If you have not been trained in CPR or are hesitant to perform ventilations, for any reason—don't give up. Your actions can still save a life.

Compression only CPR is CPR without mouth-to-mouth breaths. Provide high quality chest compressions by pushing hard and fast on the centre of the chest, at a rate of about 100 times per minute.

This potentially lifesaving option can be used by people not trained in conventional CPR, or those who are unsure of their ability.

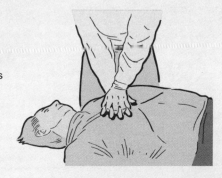

How to take over
CPR from another rescuer

CPR can be tiring. In order to maintain the most effective compressions it is recommended that rescuers switch after every 5 cycles of compressions and ventilations (approx 2 minutes).

1

Ask if you can help

Find out if medical help has been called

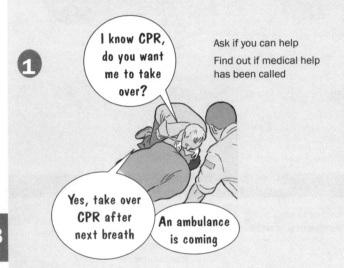

2

Give 30 compressions

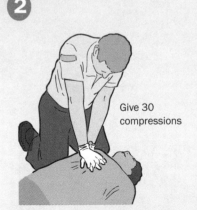

3

Gve two breaths

Continue CPR with cycles of 30 compressions and two ventilations

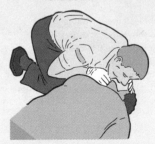

Don't use the same face shield as the first rescuer

Automated External Defibrillation—AED

Automated external defibrillation, the application of an electric shock to a heart that has stopped beating, has been proven to be one of the most important tools in saving the lives of sudden cardiac arrest casualties.

Cardiac Conduction System

4

The heart has very specialized cells that generate electrical impulses. These impulses are what cause the heart to have a rhythmic pumping action. They cause the atria and ventricles to contract and relax thereby allowing blood into the heart and forcing it out to circulate throughout the body.

The impulse begins in an area in the atria called the sinoatrial node. This area of the heart is also known as the pacemaker for it is the master electrical controller. From here the impulse travels through the atria to another node called the atrioventricular node where it then travels through the ventricles. This wave of electricity as it passes through the heart can be measured and this is what is seen on an electrocardiogram or ECG.

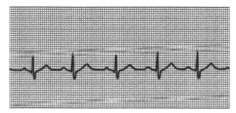

Normal ECG

When a person has a heart attack or other cardiac event, depending on how much of the heart muscle is damaged, these electrical impulses can be disturbed and the rhythm can become very chaotic. Four different types of abnormal rhythms are important to understand when learning about AEDs.

Ventricular Fibrillation (VF)—VF is the most common rhythm seen in cardiac arrest casualties. Instead of beating in a strong regular fashion, the heart quivers much like a bowl of jelly. As a result the heart is not able to pump blood to the body and the casualty will not have a pulse. Ventricular fibrillation, if not corrected, will result in death.

ECG–
Ventricular
Fibrillation
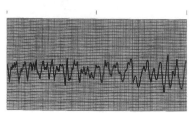

4

Pulseless Ventricular Tachycardia (VT)—This is a very fast heart rate (above 180 beats per minute) that also interferes with the pumping action of the heart. VT without a pulse is a life- threatening rhythm and like VF must be corrected as soon as possible.

ECG–Ventricular
Tachycardia
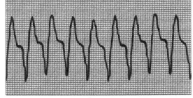

Asystole—Asystole is a condition in which there is no electrical activity in the heart at all, the "flat line" on an ECG.

Pulseless Electrical Activity (PEA)—In PEA you would see what looks like a normal heart rhythm on the ECG. In fact there is no pulse. This often occurs in trauma casualties where so much blood is lost that the heart is pumping but there is no fluid left to pump.

It is important to know about these last two rhythms because AEDs will not shock asystole or PEA.

How Do AEDs Work?

An AED is an electronic device that is programmed to recognize and shock two types of heart rhythms, VF and pulseless VT. If the machine recognizes either VT or VF in a casualty it will charge and will indicate, usually by a voice prompt, that a shock is advised. The purpose of this shock is to correct the abnormal electrical disturbance and reestablish the heart rhythm.

It is important to remember that AEDs will only shock when VT or VF is present. You cannot shock a heart that is in normal rhythm, nor will the machine shock asystole or PEA.

Time — The Crucial Factor

Time is a critical factor in determining survival from cardiac arrest. CPR should be started immediately to help prevent brain damage. Defibrillation must also be p erfomed early to be most effective. The reason for this is that the heart will only stay in fibrillation a short time before all electrical activity ceases. Quick defibrillation means more heart muscle saved in cardiac arrest casualties. Studies have shown that for each minute that defibrillation is delayed, the chance of survival declines by up to ten percent. Few cardiac arrest casualties survive if defibrillation is delayed longer than twelve minutes.

The Role of CPR in AED

In most cases CPR alone will not restart the heart. It is however an important link in the Chain of Survival™. Not only does it keep oxygenated blood flowing to the brain, it also helps extend the length of time that the heart will remain in VT or VF. This is important because these are the only types of rhythms that AEDs will shock. CPR then can "buy some time" for the casualty until the AED is attached and ready to deliver a shock.

Using an AED (always follow the manufacturer's instructions)

1   Press the POWER ON button.

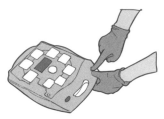

2   Connect cables to AED.

3   Attach cables to electrode pads (with some models both are pre-connected.) Attach adhesive electrode pads to the casualty's chest.

4   Bare the chest. Shave the chest if very hairy chest. Dry the chest if wet. Pads adhere better to a smooth, dry surface.

Peel away the protective plastic and attach electrode pads — one pad on the right upper anterior side of the casualty's chest just below the collarbone and one pad on the left lower anterior chest wall just below the nipple. Some electrodes have instructions on where they should be placed.

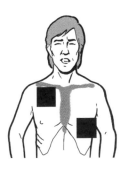

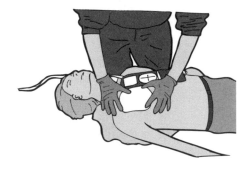

5   Stand back and ensure no one is touching the casualty (clear casualty).

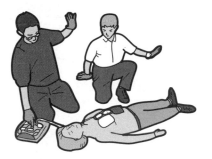

6   Press the ANALYZE button on the defibrillator and follow the voice prompts (some machines automatically analyze when the pads are applied).

Once the machine has analyzed the heart rhythm it will indicate either shock required or no shock required.

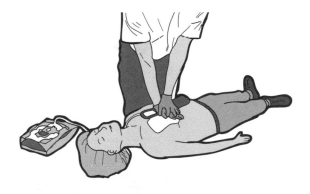

4

AED Shock/No Shock Algorithm

Assess/analyze

Shockable rhythm

Shock

Non-shockable rhythm

No shock

CPR for 2 minutes (5 cycles)

Post-resuscitation care and handover to EMS

If defibrillation is successful, the casualty may start breathing on his own but remain unresponsive. In this case place the casualty into the recovery position and monitor the ABCs. Leave the AED attached. Some machines continually monitor heart rhythms or you may need to use the device if the casualty's heart stops again.

Certain information is important for emergency services personnel such as the time of collapse, time when CPR was started, time when first shock was delivered and number of shocks. Provide as much detail as possible and follow the directions of medical personnel once they arrive on the scene.

4

Defibrillation—Special Considerations and Special Circumstances

The following are important considerations to be aware of when using these devices.

AEDs in pregnant patients—AEDs can be used in all stages of pregnancy.

AEDs and pacemakers or implanted defibrillators—Some people have pacemakers implanted under their skin to help the heart maintain a normal rhythm. Defibrillator pads should not be placed directly over the pacemaker site but should be approximately one inch away. Similarly, other people have a small defibrillator implanted under their skin which will automatically deliver a shock to the heart if VF or VT is detected. Again you should not place your defibrillator pads over the implanted device. Look for scars on the chest as an indicator of implanted devices. If you see minor contractions in the chest area while you are getting ready to defibrillate, wait 20-30 seconds until the casualty's implanted defibrillator is finished. You can touch the casualty while his implanted defibrillator is shocking without danger to yourself.

AEDs and children—Automated external defibrillators (AEDs) may be used for children and infants. For these younger casualties, the device should deliver a pediatric adjusted energy level usually through the use of special pads or a setting on the machine. The device should be highly specific for pediatric shockable rhythms either VF or VT. If you do not have a device with pediatric pads or which has settings for pediatric casualties use adult pads. Some adult pads show an alternate placement for children/infants. Do not use pediatric pads on casualties over the age of 8. Use adult pads and settings in this situation.

AEDs in trauma casualties—AEDs are not recommended for patients who have suffered severe traumatic injuries. However, traumatic injuries may not always look severe or may look more severe then they actually are. In cardiac arrest where trauma is suspected, the rescuer should assess the ABCs and administer CPR and use an AED as required. Once the patient is stabilized, trauma injuries should be assessed and treated. Rapid transport to a trauma center is highly recommended

AEDs and hypothermic casualties—In the severely hypothermic casualty, use the standard shock/no shock algorithm.

AEDs and patch medications—Some casualties wear a patch that contains medication such as nitroglyercin for angina. If you see a patch gently remove it from the chest and wipe the area clean. Handle the patch carefully to avoid being affected yourself by the medication.

AEDs in a wet environment—Because AEDs generate electricity, you need to be careful in wet environments. Move the casualty to a dry area if possible and wipe the chest with a towel or cloth. If you or the casualty is submersed in water, avoiding using an AED.

AEDs on metal surfaces—It is best if casualties are on non-conductive surfaces but you should not be at risk if you have to use a device on a casualty who is on a metal surface.

AEDs in moving vehicles—If you are transporting a casualty who is connected to an AED, stop the vehicle if you need to use the device. Sometimes, the motion of the vehicle can trick the AED into thinking that VT or VF is present and it may advise a shock when it is not needed.

4

AED Troubleshooting and Maintenance

Sometimes the device will indicate "Check Electrodes". If this occurs, check the cable to pads connection, the cable to machine connection and the adherence of the pads to the casualty's chest particularly if the casualty has a very hairy chest or if the chest was wet prior to attaching the pads.

Machines will also advise if motion is detected or if the battery is low. AEDs are sold with an instruction manual that will outline troubleshooting in detail.

While AEDs are becoming easier to use and maintain, regular maintenance and operational checks are required and will help avoid problems when you have to use the device on a casualty. Follow the manufacturer's suggested schedule and checklist.

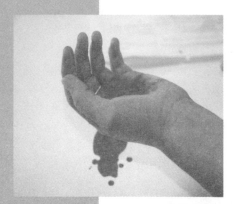

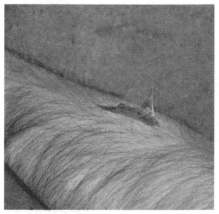

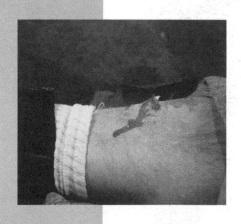

CHAPTER

5

WOUNDS AND BLEEDING

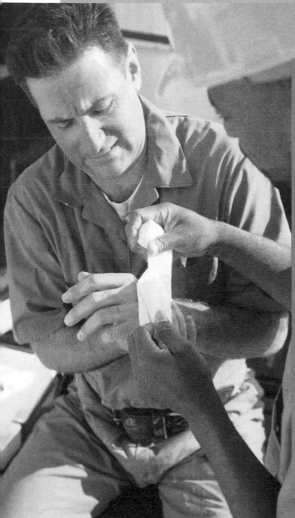

- ◆ *Dressings and bandages*
- ◆ *Slings*
- ◆ *Types of wounds*
- ◆ *First aid for severe external bleeding*
- ◆ *First aid for internal bleeding*
- ◆ *Amputations*
- ◆ *Head and facial injuries*
- ◆ *Eye injuries*
- ◆ *Chest injuries*
- ◆ *Abdominal injuries*
- ◆ *Burns*
- ◆ *Bites and stings*

Dressings and bandages

Dressings and bandages are the basic tools of first aid. They are essential for wound care and for the care of injuries to bones, joints and muscles. You should know how to use commercially prepared dressings and bandages, and also be ready to improvise with materials on hand at the emergency scene. Knowing what makes a good dressing and bandage helps you do this.

Dressings

5

A dressing is a protective covering put on a wound to help control bleeding, absorb blood from the wound, and prevent further contamination. A dressing should be:

◆ sterile, or as clean as possible

◆ large enough to completely cover the wound

◆ highly absorbent to keep the wound dry

◆ compressible, thick and soft—especially for severe bleeding so that pressure is applied evenly over the wound

◆ non-stick and lint-free to reduce the possibility of sticking to the wound—gauze, cotton and linen make good dressings; wool or other fluffy materials make poor dressings

Dressings are available in a variety of sizes and designs. The dressings used most often in first aid are:

◆ adhesive dressings—prepared sterile gauze dressings with their own adhesive strips. They are sealed in a paper or plastic covering and are available in various sizes and shapes, according to their intended use. They are often used for minor wounds with minimal bleeding

♦ gauze dressings—in varying sizes, folded and
packaged individually or in large numbers—
packaged gauze is usually sterile

♦ pressure dressings—sterile dressings of gauze and
other absorbent material, usually with an attached
roller bandage. They are used to apply pressure to a
wound with severe bleeding

♦ improvised dressings—prepared from lint-free sterile
or clean material, preferably white. They may be
made from a towel, a sheet, a pillow slip or any
other clean absorbent material such as a sanitary
pad. Plastic wrap or the wrapping from a sterile
dressing can be used as an airtight dressing for
penetrating wounds of the chest

Follow the guidelines below for putting on dressings:

♦ prevent further contamination as much as you can—
use the cleanest material available as dressings, and
wear gloves or wash your hands before handling
them (see page 173) for more on preventing further
contamination

♦ extend the dressing beyond the edges of the wound
to completely cover it

♦ if blood soaks through a dressing, leave it in place
and cover with more dressings

♦ secure a dressing with tape or bandages

Bandages

A bandage is any material that is used to hold a dressing
in place, maintain pressure over a wound, support a limb
or joint, immobilize parts of the body or secure a splint.
Bandages may be commercially prepared or improvised.

When using bandages, remember to:

◆ apply them firmly to make sure bleeding is controlled or immobilization is achieved

◆ check the circulation beyond the bandage frequently to ensure the bandage is not too tight

◆ use your bandages only as bandages, not as padding or dressings, when other materials are available— you may need all your bandages for other injuries

The triangular bandage

One of the most versatile prepared or improvised bandages is the triangular bandage. It is made by cutting a one-metre square of linen or cotton on the diagonal, producing two triangles. Triangular bandages can be improvised from sheets, garbage bags, canvas, etc. The parts of the triangular bandage are:

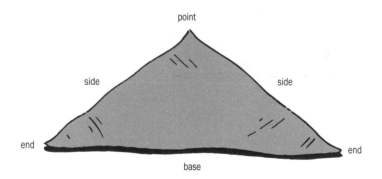

point

side   side

end   end

base

A triangular bandage may be used:

♦ as a whole cloth—opened to its fullest extent, as a sling or to hold a large dressing in place

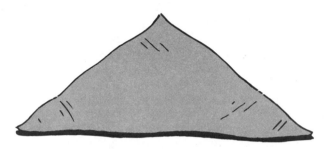

♦ as a broad bandage—to hold splints in place or to apply pressure evenly over a large area

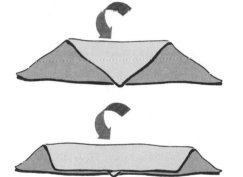

Fold the point to the centre of the base with the point slightly beyond the base

Fold in half again from the top to the base

♦ as a narrow bandage—to secure dressings or splints or to immobilize ankles and feet in a figure-8

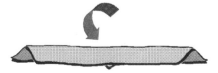

Fold a broad bandage in half again from the top to the base

5

Using a triangular bandage to hold a dressing in place

The following bandages are useful for holding dressings or padding in place. The instructions that follow use a full triangular bandage, but this may be too large in some cases. For a smaller casualty, fold a triangular bandage in half, end-to-end, to make a smaller triangular bandage.

5

Reef knot—the knot of choice

The reef knot is the best knot for tying bandages and slings because:

◆ it lies flat, making it more comfortable than other knots

◆ it doesn't slip

◆ it is easy to untie

To tie a reef knot:

◆ take one end of a bandage in each hand

◆ lay the end from the right hand over the one from the left hand and pass it under to form a half-knot. This will transfer the ends from one hand to the other

◆ the end now in the left hand should be laid over the one from the right and passed under to form another half-knot. The finished knot looks like two intertwined loops

◆ tighten by pulling one loop against the other or by pulling only on the ends

Place knots so they do not cause discomfort by pressing on skin or bone, particularly at the site of a fracture or at the neck, when tying a sling.

If the knot is uncomfortable, place soft material underneath as padding.

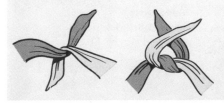

Head bandage

1   Stand behind the casualty. Use a triangular
bandage as a whole cloth with a narrow hem
folded along the base. Place the centre of the
base in the middle of the forehead, close to
the eyebrows.

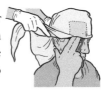

2   Bring the point over the top of the head to
cover the dressing, and down the back of the
head. Bring the ends around the back of the
head, cross over the point, and around the
head to the front. Tie the ends together, using
a reef knot, low on the forehead.

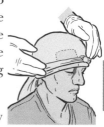

3   Steady the head with one hand, and gently
pull the point down to put the desired
amount of pressure on the dressing. Fold
the point up toward the top of the head and
secure it carefully with a safety pin or tuck it
under the back crisscross.

Knee or elbow bandage

1   Use a triangular bandage as a whole cloth with
a narrow hem folded along the base. Place the
centre of the base on the leg below the kneecap with
the point toward the top of the leg (or to bandage
an elbow, on the forearm with the point toward the
shoulder).

2   Bring the ends around the joint,
crossing over the point in front of the
elbow or at the back of the knee. Pad
under the knot if possible.

3 Bring the ends up and tie off over the point. Pull the point up to put the right amount of pressure on the dressing and then fold it down and secure it with a safety pin or tuck it under the knot.

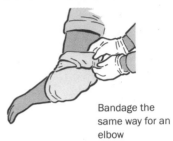

Pull on the point to put pressure on the dressing

Bandage the same way for an elbow

5

Foot or hand bandage

1 Use a triangular bandage as a whole cloth. Place it on a flat surface with the point away from the casualty.

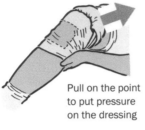

2 Place the foot or hand on the triangular bandage with the toes or fingers toward the point, leaving enough bandage at the ankle or wrist to fully cover the part. Bring the point up and over the foot or hand to rest on the lower leg or wrist.

3 Bring the ends alongside the foot or hand and crisscross the folded ends up and around the ankle or wrist. Cross over the point and wrap any extra bandage before tying it off.

4 Tie off over the point. If the point extends beyond the knot, pull it up to apply the desired pressure. Fold it downward and tuck under the knot.

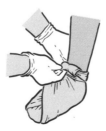

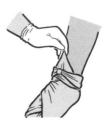

Roller bandage

Roller bandages, usually made of gauze-like material, are packaged as a roll. Use them to hold dressings in place or to secure splints.

Put on a roller bandage in a simple spiral. Starting at the narrow part of the limb, anchor the bandage as follows:

◆ place the end of the bandage on a diagonal at the starting point

◆ wrap the bandage around the injured part so the corner of the bandage end is left out

5

◆ fold this corner of the bandage over and wrap the bandage around again to cover the corner

Continue wrapping the bandage, overlapping each turn by one quarter to one third of the bandage's width. Make full-width overlaps with the final two or three turns and secure with a safety pin, adhesive tape or by cutting and tying the bandage as shown. Check circulation below the bandage.

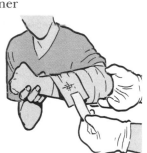

Tubular gauze and elasticized net bandages

When bleeding has been controlled and direct pressure is not required, quick and efficient bandaging can be accomplished with tubular gauze or elasticized net bandages. Both types of bandage come in various sizes to fit different parts of the body. Cut the required length from the roll and either apply it with a specially-designed applicator or stretch it by hand to fit over the dressing.

Apply roller bandages firmly, but not too tightly. Check circulation below the injury after putting on the bandage. Check it again every few minutes—as the injured part swells, circulation could be cut off.

Tubular gauze and elasticized net are especially useful for holding dressings to the head, shoulder, thigh or finger where roller bandaging is difficult and time-consuming. Instructions on how to put them on are usually included with the bandage.

Figure-8

A figure-8 bandage is used to tie the ankles and feet, to secure a splint to the ankles/feet, or to support an injured ankle.

To tie a figure-8:

◆ position the centre of a narrow or broad triangular bandage under the ankle (or both ankles if tying the feet together). The bandage may be positioned over a dressing or splint

◆ bring the ends around the ankles, cross over on top of the legs and bring the ends around the feet

◆ tie the figure-8 off where the knot will not put pressure on the foot—either between the feet or on the sole of the shoe

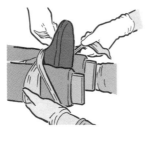 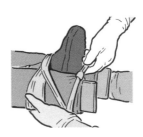

Slings

A sling provides support and protection for an arm. Commercial slings are available, but a sling can be easily improvised with a scarf, belt, necktie or other item that can go around the casualty's neck—any material will do as long as it is sturdy enough to support the arm. You can also support the arm by placing the hand inside a buttoned jacket or by pinning the sleeve of a shirt or jacket to the clothing in the proper position.

Arm sling

The arm sling is used to support an injured elbow, forearm, wrist or hand . To put on an arm sling:

1   Support the forearm of the injured limb across the body, with the wrist and hand slightly higher than the elbow. Place an open triangular bandage between the forearm and the chest so the point extends beyond the elbow and the base is straight up and down.

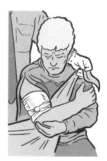

2   Bring the upper end over the casualty's shoulder on the uninjured side, around the back of the neck to the front of the injured side. While still supporting the forearm, bring the lower end of the bandage over the hand and forearm and tie off on the injured side in the hollow of the collarbone. Place padding under the knot for comfort.

3   Bring the point around to the front of the elbow and secure with a safety pin, or twist the point into a "pigtail" and tuck it inside the sling.

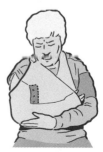

4   Adjust the sling so you can see the fingernails—this way you can watch them to check on circulation.

St. John tubular sling

Use a St. John tubular sling to support the hand and forearm in a well-elevated position that transfers the weight of the arm and hand to the uninjured side. This sling is used for injuries to the shoulder or collarbone, and for bleeding of the hand. To put on a St. John tubular sling:

5

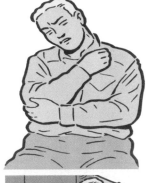

1 Support the forearm of the injured side diagonally across the chest, with the fingers pointing toward the opposite shoulder.

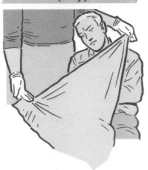

2 Place a triangular bandage over the forearm and hand with the point extending beyond the elbow and the upper end over the shoulder on the uninjured side.

The base is placed vertically in line with the body on the uninjured side.

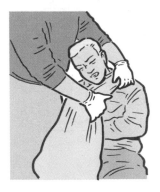

3 Support the forearm and ease the base of the bandage under the hand, forearm and elbow. Tuck the base of the bandage under the injured arm to make a pocket that runs the full length of the arm.

4   Gather the bandage at the elbow and bring the lower end across the back and over the shoulder on the uninjured side.

To gather the bandage, twist it around and around towards the body—this closes the pocket at the elbow.

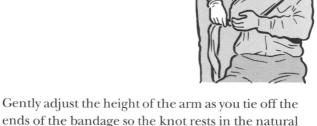

5   Gently adjust the height of the arm as you tie off the ends of the bandage so the knot rests in the natural hollow above the collarbone. Place padding under knot, if available.

Tie the sling tightly enough to support the weight of the injured arm.

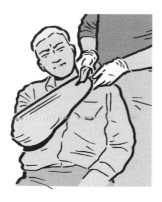

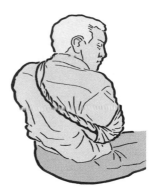

Wounds and bleeding

A wound is any break in the soft tissues of the body. It usually results in bleeding and may allow germs to enter the body. Bleeding is the escape of blood from the blood vessels into surrounding tissues, body cavities or out of the body. The soft tissues of the body are the most susceptible to injury, resulting in wounds and bleeding.

A wound can be either open or closed:

5

◆ **open wound**—there is a break in the outer layer of the skin that results in bleeding and may permit germs to enter the body, causing infection

◆ **closed wound**—there is no break in the outer layer of skin so there is no external bleeding (but there will be internal bleeding which may be severe) and the risk of infection is low (except in a closed abdominal wound where the risk of infection is high—see page 191).

Different types of wounds are described on page 169. When someone is injured, recognizing the type of wound helps to give appropriate first aid.

The aim in the care of wounds is to stop the bleeding and prevent infection. Although some bleeding may help to wash contamination from the wound, excessive blood flow must be stopped quickly to minimize shock.

Types of wounds

Contusions or bruises

Contusions or bruises are closed wounds usually caused by a fall or a blow from something blunt. The tissues under the skin are damaged and bleed into surrounding tissues, causing discolouration. Because there is no break in the skin, there is little chance of infection. A bruise may be a sign of a deeper, more serious injury or illness.

Lacerations

Lacerations are tears in the skin and underlying tissue. The edges of the wound are jagged and irregular, and dirt is likely to be present, increasing the risk of infection. Lacerations are often caused by machinery, barbed wire or the claws of an animal.

Abrasions or scrapes

Abrasions or scrapes are open wounds where the outer protective layer of skin and the tiny underlying blood vessels are exposed. The deeper layer of the skin is still intact. Examples of abrasions include rug burn and road rash. Abrasions do not bleed very much but can be very painful. The risk of infection is high.

Puncture wounds

Puncture wounds are open wounds caused by blunt or pointed instruments, such as knives, nails or an animal's teeth. The wound may have a small opening, but often penetrates deep into the tissue. There may be contamination deep in the wound and internal organs may be damaged.

Incisions

Incisions are clean cuts in soft tissue caused by something sharp such as a knife. These wounds may not be as dirty as abrasions, but they may contain fragments of glass or other material.

Avulsions and Amputations

Avulsions are injuries that leave a piece of skin or other tissue either partially or completely torn away from the body. Amputations involve partial or complete loss of a body part and are usually caused by machinery or cutting tools.

> ⚠ Gunshot wounds are a special type of wound. The entry wound is often small, and may have burns around it. Sometimes there is an exit wound as well, which is usually larger than the entry wound. Because the bullet may bounce around inside the body, the exit wound may not be directly across from the entry wound.

5

Bleeding

Bleeding is the escape of blood from the blood vessels. In external bleeding, blood escapes the body through a surface wound—you can see external bleeding.

In internal bleeding, blood escapes from tissues inside the body—you don't usually see internal bleeding. Also, bleeding is either arterial, which is bleeding from the arteries, or venous, which is bleeding from the veins.

Signs and symptoms of external bleeding

In **arterial bleeding**, the blood is bright red and spurts with each heartbeat—arterial bleeding is serious and often hard to control

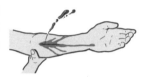

In **venous bleeding**, the blood is dark red and flows more steadily—it is easier to stop than arterial bleeding

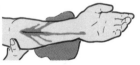

The most obvious sign of external bleeding is blood. You do not always see blood with internal bleeding. General signs and symptoms of bleeding vary depending on how much blood is lost. Severe blood loss will result in the following signs and symptoms of shock:

- ◆ pale, cold and clammy skin

- ◆ rapid pulse, gradually becoming weaker

- ◆ faintness, dizziness, thirst and nausea

- ◆ restlessness and apprehension

- ◆ shallow breathing, yawning, sighing and gasping for air

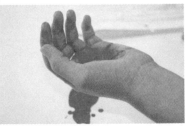

First aid for severe external bleeding

The principles for preventing further contamination and first aid for bleeding are on pages 173 and 174. The following sequence shows the principles being used.

1 Begin ESM—do a scene survey. Assess the mechanism of injury. If you suspect a head or spinal injury, steady and support the head and neck before continuing.

2 Do a primary survey and give first aid for life-threatening injuries.

3 To control severe bleeding, apply direct pressure to the wound as quickly as possible. If the wound is large and wide open, you may have to bring the edges of the wound together first.

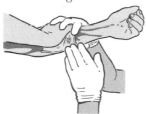

4 Place the casualty at rest—this will further reduce blood flow and will reduce the risk of injury if the casualty becomes dizzy or faints.

5 Quickly replace the casualty's hand with dressings (preferably sterile) and continue direct pressure over the dressings.

6 Once bleeding is under control, continue the primary survey, looking for other life-threatening injuries. Give life-saving first aid as needed.

7 Before bandaging the wound, check circulation below the injury.

8 Bandage the dressing in place.

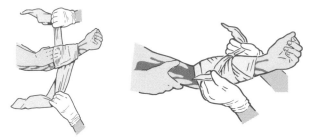

9 Check the circulation below the injury and compare it with the other side. If it is worse than it was before the injury was bandaged, loosen the bandage just enough to improve circulation.

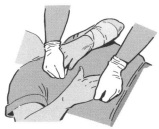

10 Give ongoing casualty care, including first aid to minimize shock (see page 67).

If the dressings become blood-soaked, don't remove them—add more dressings and continue pressure. Removing the blood-soaked dressings may disturb blood clots and expose the wound to further contamination.

Preventing further contamination

All open wounds are contaminated to some degree. From the moment of injury, there is risk of infection that continues until the wound is completely healed. Stopping bleeding is your priority, but do it using the cleanest materials available.

Minor wound care

Follow the principles listed below for cleaning a wound. Tell the casualty to seek medical help if signs of infection appear later.

◆ wash your hands with soap and water and put on gloves if available

◆ do not cough or breathe directly over the wound

◆ fully expose the wound but don't touch it

◆ gently wash loose material from the surface of the wound. Wash and dry the surrounding skin with clean dressings, wiping away from the wound. An antibiotic cream can be used on superficial wounds and abrasions

◆ cover the wound promptly with a sterile dressing. Tape the dressing in place

◆ remove and dispose of gloves in an appropriate manner (see page 18) and wash your hands and any other skin area that may have been in contact with the casualty's blood

Wound infection

Any wound that becomes infected should be seen by a doctor.

Use the acronym SHARP to identify signs and symptoms of infection.

Recognize infection in a wound when the wound:

S—becomes **SWOLLEN**

H—obvious **HEAT** as the injured area feels warmer than the surrounding area

A—becomes painful or **ACHES**

R—becomes **RED**

P—shows the presence of **PUS** (whitish fluid)

5

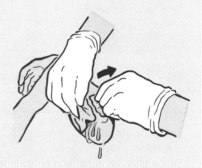

Tetanus Infection

Any wound may be contaminated by spores that cause tetanus, a potentially fatal disease characterized by muscle spasms. Tetanus is commonly referred to as "lockjaw."

Deep wounds, especially those caused by animal bites or those that may have been contaminated by soil, dust or animal feces, are at high risk of tetanus infection. Advise a casualty with this type of wound to get medical help.

Principles of controlling bleeding

The body has natural defences against bleeding. Damaged blood vessels constrict to reduce blood flow and blood pressure drops as bleeding continues. These factors result in reduced force of blood flow. Blood will clot as it is exposed to air, forming a seal at the wound. Even so, the first aider should try to stop all bleeding as soon as possible, following the ABC priorities.

Steps to control bleeding

The following steps will control all but the most severe bleeding—you can often do these all at the same time.

Direct pressure—apply pressure directly to the wound to stop blood flow and allow clots to form. When bleeding is controlled, keep the pressure on the wound with dressings and bandages.

Rest—place the casualty at rest to reduce the pulse rate. Unless the bleeding is from a head wound, the preferred position is lying down.

Minor cuts and scrapes that cause slight bleeding are easily controlled with pressure, and rest. Severe bleeding must be brought under control quickly to prevent further blood loss and to slow the progress of shock.

Wound closures

Wound closures are special adhesive strips used to bring wound edges together to assist healing. For small gaping wounds without complications, wound closures may eliminate the need for stitches.

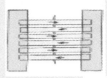

Transparent strip closures

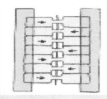

Butterfly closures

Commercially prepared adhesive dressings

Commercially prepared adhesive dressings combine the dressing, padding and bandage all in one and are available in a variety of shapes and sizes.

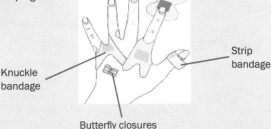

Fingertip bandage

Strip bandage

Knuckle bandage

Butterfly closures

Checking
circulation below an injury

Causes of impaired circulation

Certain injuries and first aid procedures may impair (reduce or cut off) circulation to the tissue below the injury (called distal circulation). A joint

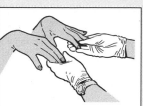

injury or fracture could pinch an artery and restrict the flow of blood to the limb. Bandages tied too tightly will impair distal circulation. Sometimes, a bandage is not too tight when it is put on but as the injury swells, the bandage becomes too tight, impairing circulation.

Effects of impaired circulation

If oxygenated blood does not reach the tissues below the injury, there may be tissue damage that could lead to loss of the limb. Check circulation below an injury before tying any bandages. Check again after tying bandages. If circulation is impaired, take steps to improve it.

How to monitor circulation

For each of the methods below, check both the injured side and the uninjured side of the casualty. If circulation is not impaired, both sides will be the same. Monitor circulation below the injury by:

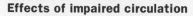

◆ checking skin colour—if the skin does not have full colour, circulation may be impaired

◆ checking skin temperature—if the skin temperature feels cold, especially if it is colder than the uninjured side, circulation may be impaired

◆ checking for a pulse—in an arm injury, check for a pulse at the wrist

◆ doing the nailbed test—press on a fingernail or toenail until the nailbed turns white, and then release it. Note how long it takes for normal colour to return. If it returns quickly, blood flow is unrestricted. If it stays white, or if the colour returns slowly, circulation may be impaired

When the injury is on the arm, expose the hands and fingers to check circulation. When the injury is on the leg and there is no reason to remove the shoe, check circulation by placing fingers inside the sock along the side of the foot.

Improving impaired circulation

To improve impaired circulation, loosen tight bandages. If circulation doesn't improve and medical help will be delayed, try moving the limb to restore circulation. By moving the limb, you will hopefully relieve any pressure on blood vessels. If possible, move the limb towards its natural position. Only move the limb as much as the casualty will let you, or as far as you can without resistance. Resecure the limb and recheck circulation.

Keep monitoring circulation until medical help takes over. If circulation remains impaired, medical help is urgently needed.

5

Recognizing internal bleeding

Internal bleeding may not be easy to recognize—a casualty can bleed to death without any blood being seen. Suspect internal bleeding if:

◆ the casualty received a severe blow or a penetrating injury to the chest, neck, abdomen or groin

◆ there are major limb fractures such as a fractured upper leg or pelvis

◆ the mechanism of injury suggests internal injury is likely (e.g. excessive force to the body from a car crash)

Specific signs of internal bleeding

You may recognize internal bleeding by one or more of the following characteristic signs. Blood is:

◆ coming from the ear canal or the nose, or it may appear as a bloodshot eye or black eye (bleeding inside the head)

◆ coughed up and looks bright red and frothy (bleeding into the lungs)

◆ seen in vomitus either as bright red, or brown like coffee grounds

◆ seen in the stools, and looks either black and tarry (bleeding into the upper bowel), or its normal red colour (bleeding into the lower bowel)

◆ seen in the urine as a red or smoky brown colour (bleeding into the urinary tract)

◆ signs of shock without external injury

If internal bleeding is severe, the casualty will show progressive signs of shock.

First aid for severe, internal bleeding

As a first aider, you can do very little to control internal bleeding. Give first aid to minimize shock and get medical help as quickly as you can.

1   Begin ESM—do a scene survey.

2   Do a primary survey and give first aid for life-threatening injuries. If the mechanism of injury suggests a severe blow to the body, look further for signs of internal bleeding.

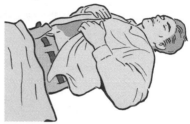

Place the casualty in the shock position (see page 68).

3   Send or go for medical help.

4   Give ongoing casualty care. Do not give the casualty anything by mouth. If he complains of thirst, moisten his lips with a wet cloth. Make the casualty comfortable—loosen all tight clothing at the neck, chest and waist. Keep the casualty warm and protected from extreme temperatures.

Monitor the casualty often. When medical help takes over, tell them you suspect internal bleeding.

Amputations

An amputation is when a part of the body, such as a toe, foot or leg, has been partly or completely cut off. When this happens, you must control the bleeding from the wound, care for the amputated tissue and get medical help. The first aid for both a completely amputated hand and a partly amputated finger is shown below.

First aid for amputations

1   Begin ESM—do a scene survey. Do a primary survey and give first aid for life-threatening injuries. In this case, there is severe bleeding from an amputation.

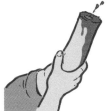

2   Control the bleeding—apply direct pressure to the wound. Reposition a partly amputated part to its normal position.

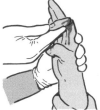

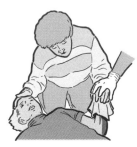

Do not try to clean an amputated part.

Do not use any antiseptic solutions.

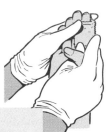

Apply direct pressure and cover the area with thick sterile gauze that is moistened, if possible

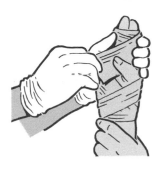 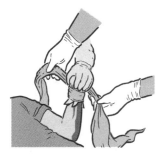

3 Send for medical help and give ongoing casualty care to the casualty, including first aid for shock.

4 Care for the amputated tissue—completely or partly amputated parts must be preserved, regardless of their condition, and taken to medical help with the casualty. It may be possible to reattach the part—and with the proper care of the part, the chances are even better.

Care for the amputated part by wrapping the amputated part in a clean, moist dressing—if you can't moisten the dressing, a dry dressing will do.

5 Keep the amputated part in a shaded, cool place and get the casualty and the amputated part to medical help as soon as possible.

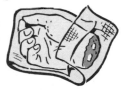

Put the amputated part in a clean, watertight plastic bag and seal it.

Put this bag in a second plastic bag or container partly filled with crushed ice.

Attach a record of the date and time this was done and send this package with the casualty to medical help.

General first aid for hand and foot injuries

Hand and foot injuries are common. The following are first aid guidelines for these injuries:

1   Begin ESM—do a scene survey. Expose and assess the injury.

2   Give first aid for any severe bleeding—direct pressure, and rest (see page 171).

3   Remove any jewellery before swelling occurs.

4   For wounds without severe bleeding, brush away loose debris and cover with dressings. If there are wounds on the fingers or toes, put dressings, preferably non-stick dressings, between the fingers and toes to prevent them from sticking together.

5   If there are signs of fractures, or if there is any significant loss of function, immobilize the hand or foot as shown on pages 268 and 279.

6   Get medical help.

If the injury seems minor, such as a minor sprain or minor wound, and the casualty chooses not to get medical help, tell him that within 48 hours it should be obvious that the injury is well on the way to healing. If this is not the case, and there is still pain, loss of function, or perhaps an infection, tell the casualty he should get medical help to ensure there are no complications and that everything is being done to ensure a full recovery.

First aid for bleeding from the palm of the hand

1 Start ESM—do a scene survey. Do a primary survey and give first aid for life-threatening injuries. In this case, there is severe bleeding from a wound to the hand. Expose the wound.

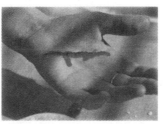

2 Control the bleeding—apply direct pressure. The casualty can use his other hand to apply direct pressure while you locate a first aid kit. Bandage dressings in place.

Put a dressing over the wound and fill the palm with more dressings or a bulky pad. Check the circulation in the fingers and compare it with the other hand.

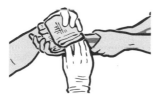

Bend the fingers over the pad to make a fist and bandage the hand so the fist is held firmly closed.

3 Place the middle of a narrow triangular bandage on the inside of the wrist and bring the ends around the back of the hand.

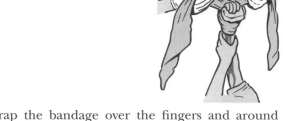

Wrap the bandage over the fingers and around the wrist tightly, but not so tight as to cut off circulation.

Leave the thumb exposed, if possible, to check circulation. Tie the bandage off at the wrist and tuck in the ends

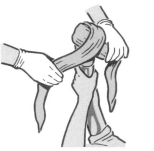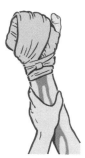

4 Support the injured hand. Use a St. John tubular sling (see page 166). Recheck the circulation below the injury.

5 Give ongoing casualty care and get medical help.

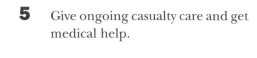

Pinched fingernail

When a finger, thumb or toe has been pinched, the pressure from the blood under the nail can cause great pain. You can relieve this pain as follows:

◆ place the injured part under cool running water to reduce pain and swelling

◆ if the pain is severe, and you can see pooled blood under the nail, release the pressure under the nail as follows:

❖ straighten a paper clip and heat one end to red hot, using a stove element or the flame from a lighter—be careful not to burn yourself

❖ place the heated end of the paper clip on top of the nail and let it burn a hole to release the pooled blood

❖ once the pressure has been released, wash the area with soap and water and put on an adhesive dressing.

5

Don't use a needle—the hole it makes is too small to release the pooled blood effectively.

 First aid for a contusion (bruise)

With a contusion or bruise, blood escapes into the surrounding tissue. Relieve the pain and reduce the swelling by following RICE (see page 238).

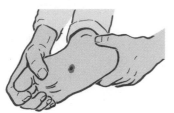

Puncture wounds

All puncture wounds must be considered serious because of the possibility of serious tissue damage and contamination deep inside the wound.

 First aid for puncture wounds

1   Begin ESM—do a scene survey and a primary survey. Wash your hands or put on gloves.

2   Start the secondary survey—expose the wound. Although there may not be much external bleeding, you should suspect internal bleeding, especially if the wound is in the chest or abdomen.

3   Control bleeding with direct pressure, (see page 174), dress the wound, and transport the casualty to medical help.

4   Give ongoing casualty care until handover.

Gunshot wounds

A gunshot wound is a special type of wound (see page 169 for more on gunshot wounds).

 First aid for gunshot wounds

The aim of first aid for gunshot wounds is to give life-saving first aid and get the casualty to medical help as quickly as possible.

1   Begin ESM—do a scene survey. If there is any possibility of danger to yourself, don't go any further. Call the police.

2 Do a primary survey and give first aid for life-threatening conditions. When looking for bleeding, examine all parts of the body very carefully. The exit wound may not be where you expect it to be—look for it carefully.

3 Place the casualty at rest and give first aid for shock. Do not give anything by mouth.

4 Give ongoing casualty care and transport the casualty to medical help as soon as possible.

Wounds with embedded objects

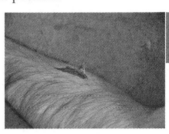

Never remove an object embedded in a wound. Removing the object will probably result in heavier bleeding and could cause further tissue damage. The aim of first aid for a wound with an embedded object is to stop the bleeding, prevent the embedded object from moving and to get medical help. The first aid is slightly different depending on whether the embedded object is short or long.

 Bandaging a wound with an embedded object

1 Wash hands or put gloves on. Expose the injured area and assess the wound.

2 To stop the bleeding, put pressure around the embedded object.

If the embedded object is short, "tent" a clean dressing loosely over the object to keep the wound clean.

3 Place bulky dressings around the object to keep it from moving. This will apply pressure to the wound but not to the object.

4   Secure the bulky material (dressings) in place with a narrow bandage, taking care that pressure is not exerted on the embedded object.

5   Check the circulation below the injury—if circulation below the injury is impaired, and it wasn't before bandaging, loosen the bandage to restore circulation. Give ongoing casualty care and get medical help.

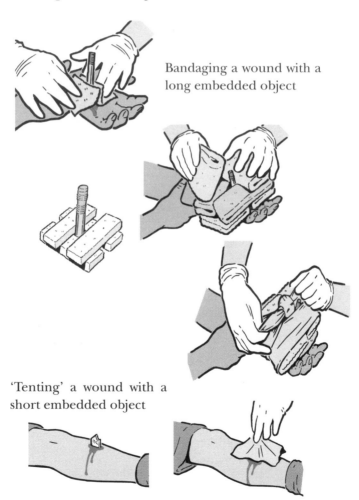

Bandaging a wound with a long embedded object

'Tenting' a wound with a short embedded object

Slivers and splinters

Slivers are embedded objects and may be wood, thorns, glass or metal. This type of injury is common in the hands and feet. Although slivers may cause discomfort and pain, in most cases they can be removed easily without complications.

In serious cases, slivers can be disabling and cause infection. Organic objects including thorns and wood slivers are particularly likely to result in infection.

Slivers should be removed if there is no threat to the surrounding tissues (the sliver is neither too large, nor embedded too deeply).

5

 Removing a sliver

1 Clean the area with soap and warm water.

2 With sterile tweezers, grip the sliver as close to the skin as possible.

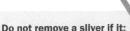

3 Pull the sliver in a straight line in the opposite direction to the angle of entry.

4 When the sliver is removed, give first aid for a puncture wound (see page 184). Get medical help if some of the sliver was not removed, there is more tissue damage than a simple, small puncture wound or if an infection develops (see page 173).

Do not remove a sliver if it:

◆ lies over a joint

◆ is deeply embedded into the flesh

◆ is in or close to the eye (see page 204)

◆ possesses a barb (e.g. metal slivers and fishhooks). This may result in tissue damage.

◆ cannot be removed easily

In these cases, give first aid for an embedded object (see page 185). Reassure the casualty and get medical help.

Chest injuries

Pneumothorax

A pneumothorax (new-mow-thor-ax) is the result of an injury where air gets into the chest cavity. Page 256 explains this in detail. Pneumothorax can cause one or both lungs to collapse, resulting in a life-threatening breathing emergency. If air is getting into the chest cavity through an open wound, the wound is called a penetrating chest wound. There may be bloodstained bubbles around the wound when the casualty exhales—these come from air being sucked into, and out of the wound as the casualty breathes (which is why these wounds are also called sucking chest wounds). First aid is needed right away.

First aid for a penetrating chest wound

1 Begin ESM—do a scene survey and primary survey. As soon as you identify a sucking chest wound, cover it by pressing the casualty's hand, a bystander's hand or your own hand over the wound (preferably a gloved hand). This stops air from flowing in and out of the chest cavity.

2 Place the casualty in the position that makes breathing easiest—this is usually semi-sitting, leaning slightly towards the injured side. This position keeps the uninjured side of the chest upward so it can be used most effectively for breathing.

3 Seal the wound with an airtight dressing taped on three sides, leaving the lowest side of the dressing open. The dressing should work as a flutter-type valve, letting air from the chest cavity out while preventing air from going into the wound. If there is an embedded object, tape dressings around the object and try to make a flutter-type valve.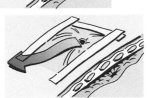

The flutter valve stops air from going into the wound by being sucked up tight against the wound when the casualty inhales

When the casualty exhales, the valve opens and allows air to exit from the chest

5

4   Assess breathing. If breathing gets worse, a tension pneumothorax may be developing (see below). If breathing is effective, go to step 5.

5   Give ongoing casualty care, monitoring breathing often.

There is not always an open wound with a pneumothorax. A pneumothorax can be caused by broken ribs, or it can happen for no obvious reason. A pneumothorax always has the potential to be a life-threatening breathing emergency and medical help is needed as quickly as possible.

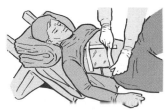 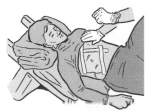

Tension pneumothorax

If breathing becomes more difficult, a tension pneumothorax may be developing. First, unseal the wound for a few seconds—air may rush out. Then adjust the dressing to make sure it seals the wound as the casualty breathes in, and unseals the wound as the casualty breathes out. You have to check this kind of dressing often to make sure it is working properly.

Blast injury

Most people never see explosives in their lifetimes. But for some Canadians, working with explosives is a way of life. This is especially true in the mining and construction industries. There are three mechanisms of injury from an explosion, apart from being right in the blast:

◆ injuries from being struck by material thrown by the blast

◆ injuries from being thrown by the blast

◆ injuries to hollow organs, including the lungs, caused by the shock wave from the blast—these can cause life-threatening breathing emergencies

The violent shock wave of an explosion can damage the lungs (and the stomach and intestines), even when there is no other visible sign of injury. The casualty may complain of chest pain and cough up frothy blood.

 First aid for a blast injury that affects breathing

1   Begin ESM—do a scene survey. If the casualty was thrown by the blast, suspect a head or spinal injury and prevent any unnecessary movement.

2   Do a primary survey. Place the casualty at rest in a semisitting position if there is no suspected head or spinal injury—raise and support the head and shoulders. Send for medical help.

3   Monitor breathing closely. If breathing stops, begin CPR with compressions (see Chapter 4).

4   Give ongoing casualty care including first aid for shock until medical help arrives.

Abdominal injuries

Abdominal wounds may be closed or open. Closed wounds occur when internal abdominal tissues are damaged but the skin is intact. Open abdominal wounds are those in which the skin has been broken. Abdominal organs may protrude out from the wound.

Complications from abdominal wounds may include severe bleeding (either internal or external) and contamination from the contents of ruptured abdominal organs. These complications may result in shock and infection.

5

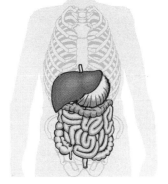

Assessing an abdominal injury

Expose the injured area. Consider the history of the incident, especially the mechanism of injury. Observe the casualty's position and examine the casualty gently. Feel for swelling, rigidity, and pain.

 ## First aid for closed abdominal wounds

If you suspect an abdominal injury, you should also suspect internal bleeding that may be severe. Give first aid for severe internal bleeding (see page 177).

First aid for open abdominal wounds

1   Begin ESM—do a scene survey. Do a primary survey. In this case you find an open abdominal wound.

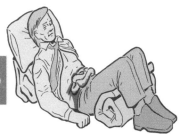

2   This wound may be open wide and must be prevented from opening wider. Position the casualty with head and shoulders slightly raised and supported, and with the knees raised.

3   Dress the wound. The method of dressing a wound of the abdominal wall depends on whether or not internal organs are protruding:

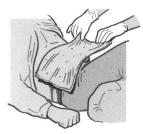

If the organs are not protruding, apply a dry dressing to the wound and bandage firmly.

If the organs are protruding, don't try to put them back into the abdomen. Put on a moist dressing as shown below. The moist dressing helps stop the organs from drying out.

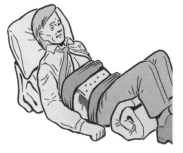

4   Do not give anything by mouth. If the casualty coughs or vomits, support the abdomen with two broad bandages.

5   Give ongoing casualty care and get the casualty to medical help promptly.

Crush injuries

"Crush injury" occurs when a portion of the body is crushed under heavy weight. The crushing force causes extensive bruising of the area, and there may be complications including fractures or ruptured organs. When the crushed area is limited, such as a hand or foot, the injury is considered serious, but is not usually life-threatening. However, a major crush injury may cause severe shock or crush syndrome, both of which are life threatening.

Severe shock can develop after a casualty is released from the weight that caused the crush injury. When the crushing force is removed, fluids from the crushed tissues leak into surrounding tissues—this causes shock.

When muscle is crushed, it releases the contents of muscle cells into the blood. If the injury is large, it can cause kidney failure. This is crush syndrome, also called post-traumatic acute renal (kidney) failure.

 First aid for crush injuries

Give first aid for wounds and fractures to stop bleeding and relieve pain. Stabilize other conditions while waiting for transportation to medical help.

1 Begin ESM—do a scene survey and a primary survey. Move the casualty as little as possible and do what you can to minimize pain.

2 Give first aid for shock right away—even if there are no signs, shock will probably develop.

3 Give ongoing casualty care and arrange transportation to medical help as soon as possible.

Head and facial injuries

First aid for a "bump on the head"

A "bump on the head" is a very common injury, especially in children. Usually it is harmless. But as with any injury to the head, it should be taken seriously—there is always the threat of an underlying skull fracture or brain injury. When a child bumps his head, do the following:

1 Begin ESM—start a scene survey. Immediately assess the mechanism of injury—was there enough force to seriously harm the child? If you think there might have been, don't move the child, and don't let him move until you check further. If the child loses consciousness, always suspect a serious injury. If you suspect a serious injury, give first aid for a head/spinal injury (see page 240).

If it appears that there is no serious injury, pick the child up and comfort him. As soon as possible, put a cold compress or ice bag (15 minutes on; 15 minutes off (see page 239)) on the injury site to relieve pain and control swelling. Watch the child for any signs or symptoms of:

♦ a skull fracture—see page 242

♦ a concussion—see page 244

♦ compression—see page 244

If you see any of these signs developing, even after many days, get medical help immediately.

Don't pick him up!

When a child falls, an adult's instinct is to pick him up and comfort him. But if there is serious injury, picking the child up could make things worse.

Don't pick up a fallen child, and don't allow a fallen child to move, until you know for sure there is no serious injury.

Bleeding from the scalp

Bleeding from the scalp is often severe and may be complicated by a fracture of the skull or an embedded object. When giving first aid for these wounds, avoid direct pressure, probing and contaminating the wound. Care must be taken to:

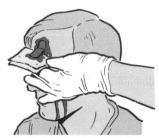

◆ clean away loose dirt

◆ apply a thick, sterile dressing that is large enough to extend well beyond the edges of the wound and bandage it firmly in place with a head bandage (see page 161)

◆ if there is suspected underlying skull fracture, give first aid for a fracture of the skull (see page 242)

◆ if there is an embedded object, apply dressings around the object to maintain pressure around but away from the wound (see page 185)

◆ give ongoing casualty care and arrange transportation of the casualty to medical aid

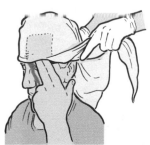

First aid for bleeding from inside the ear

1 Begin ESM—do a scene survey and assess the mechanism of injury. If you suspect a head or spinal injury, tell the casualty not to move.

2 Do a primary survey and give first aid for life-threatening conditions.

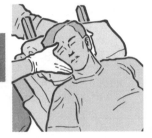

3 Do a secondary survey if needed— assess the bleeding from the ear. If the blood from the ear is mixed with straw-coloured fluid, suspect a skull fracture—steady and support the head and neck. Place a dressing lightly over the ear and give first aid for a skull fracture (see page 242). The dressing will absorb the blood and protect the wound.

4 If a head or spinal injury is not suspected, lightly tape a dressing over the ear.

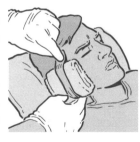

Position the casualty to allow the blood to drain from the ear if injuries permit.

If the casualty is unconscious and injuries permit, put dressings over the ear and place him in the recovery position with the injured side down.

⚠ Don't try to stop the bleeding from the ear canal by putting pressure on the ear or by packing it with dressings.

To reduce the risk of infection inside the ear, it is best to let the blood drain away.

5 Give ongoing casualty care until medical help takes over.

First aid for a nosebleed

A nosebleed may start for no obvious reason, or may be caused by blowing the nose, an injury to the nose, or in more serious cases, by an indirect injury, such as a fractured skull.

1 Begin ESM—do a scene survey and assess the mechanism of injury. If there could be a head or spinal injury, tell the casualty not to move.

2 Do a primary survey and give first aid for life-threatening conditions.

3 Assess the bleeding from the nose. If the blood from the nose is mixed with straw-coloured fluid, suspect a skull fracture. Allow the nose to bleed and give first aid for a skull fracture (see page 242).

4 If a head or spinal injury is not suspected, place the casualty in a sitting position with the head slightly forward. Leaning forward allows blood to drain from the nose and mouth instead of back into the throat.

Tell the casualty to compress the entire fleshy part below the bridge of the nose firmly with the thumb and index finger for about 10 minutes or until bleeding stops.

5 Loosen clothing around the casualty's neck and chest. Keep the casualty quiet to avoid increased bleeding. Tell the casualty to breathe through his mouth and not blow his nose for a few hours, so that blood clots will not be disturbed. If bleeding does not stop with this first aid, or if it starts again, get medical help.

Do not try to stop a nosebleed resulting from a head injury. Allow the blood to drain and get medical help.

First aid for a knocked-out tooth

A knocked-out tooth can be reimplanted if the casualty receives medical/dental help quickly.

1   Begin ESM—do a scene survey—carefully assess the mechanism of injury—was there enough force to cause a head or spinal injury?

2   Do a primary survey. Assess the airway—is there blood or swelling that could block the airway? Assess breathing and circulation and give first aid for other life-threatening conditions.

3   Apply direct pressure to stop the bleeding from the socket of the tooth.

Seat the casualty with the head forward so blood can drain out of the mouth.

4   Care for the knocked-out tooth. Place the tooth in a cup of milk. If milk is not available, the tooth may be preserved in a saline solution or wrapped in plastic wrap kept moist with the casualty's saliva. Handle the tooth by the top—don't touch the root.

Do not

◆ handle the tooth by the root

◆ try to clean an amputated part, including a knocked-out tooth. Do not use any antiseptic solutions

◆ wash out the mouth when the bleeding has stopped—this may disturb the blood clots making the injury bleed again

5   Give ongoing casualty care and get medical help. If the knocked-out tooth is the only injury, get the casualty to a dentist as quickly as possible for the best chance of reimplanting the tooth.

Bleeding from the cheek, gums or tongue

When there is bleeding from the gums or mouth, first assess the mechanism of injury to determine if there is a chance of a serious head and/or spinal injury. If so, give

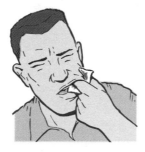

first aid for a head/spinal injury. Make sure the bleeding in the mouth doesn't block the airway.

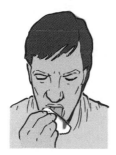

Control the bleeding in the mouth using direct pressure over a clean, preferably sterile, dressing.

Do not wash out the mouth after bleeding has stopped. This may dislodge clots and cause bleeding to start again.

Bleeding from the gums should be treated as a sign of a fractured jaw until proven otherwise (see page 243).

Wounds to the eye

Sight depends on one of the most delicate and sensitive organs of the body, the eye. The eye can be injured very easily, and for this reason, extra care must be taken to protect the eyes from hazards. When an eye is injured, proper first aid given right away may prevent partial or complete loss of eyesight.

Particles in the eye

A particle of sand, grit or a loose eyelash on the eyeball or under the eyelid causes discomfort and inflammation of the tissue around the eye. When this happens, the eye becomes a characteristic pink or reddish colour. Tears may not be enough to loosen and wash away such particles.

 To locate and remove a loose foreign particle from the eye

1   Perform a scene survey and find out what happened. If a loose particle, such as dust or an eyelash is suspected, and the particle is not sharp, the first aider should follow the procedure outlined below to locate and remove the particle.

2   Begin by asking the casualty where he feels the particle is located.

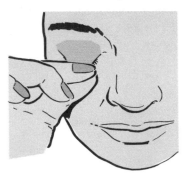

3   If it feels like the particle is under the upper lid, instruct the casualty to grasp the upper eyelashes and pull the lid straight out and then down over the lower eyelashes to try to sweep the particle away.

Try this several times. Remember to remove excess
eye make-up before attempting this procedure.

If the particle is still in the eye, try flushing it out
using clean running water from a tap, an eye cup
or eye wash bottle.

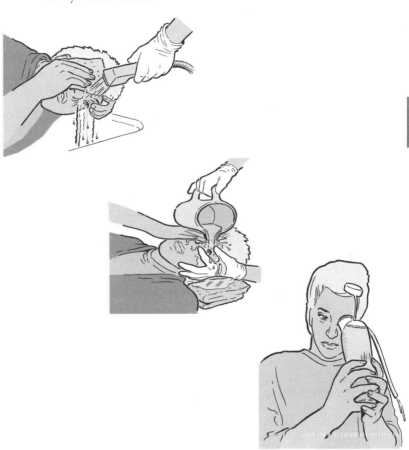

If the above methods have not been successful, you
will need to examine the surface of the eye and
under the lids.

Examining the eye

1   Wash your hands and put on gloves.

2   Seat the casualty facing a good light and steady the head.

3   With the eyes wide open and the eyelids well separated, instruct the casualty to look to the left and hold this position while you examine the other corner of the eye. A penlight will make it easier to locate the particle. When the light is directed across the eye, it will cause a shadow to appear if the particle is in the path of the light, making it easier to see.

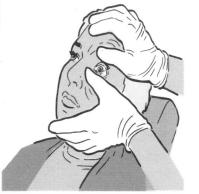

4   After examining the corners of the eye, you will need to examine under the upper and lower lids. To examine under the lower lid, gently pull down on the lower lid and ask the casualty to look up. Use your penlight to check inside the lid. To examine under the upper lid, gently pull up on the lashes and ask the casualty to look down. Use your penlight to check under the lid.

5   If you locate the particle, remove it gently using the moist corner of a facial tissue, clean cloth or cotton-tipped applicator. Do not try to remove a particle that is stuck to the eye, or is located on the coloured part of the eye.

If the casualty is wearing contact lenses, have her remove the lens before trying to remove a particle from the eye.

First aid when you cannot safely remove a particle from the eye

1   Begin ESM—do a scene survey. Wash hands or put on gloves.

2   Warn the casualty not to rub the eye because this may cause pain and tissue damage.

3   Close the casualty's eye and cover the affected eye with an eye or gauze pad. Extend the covering to the forehead and cheek to avoid pressure on the eye.

4   Secure lightly in position with a bandage or adhesive strips. Make sure there is no pressure on the eyeball.

5   Give ongoing casualty care and get medical help.

Wounds in the soft tissue around the eye

Wounds to the eyelid and soft tissue around the eye are serious because there may be injury to the eyeball. If the eyeball is not damaged, vision should not be impaired once the wounds have healed.

Blows from blunt objects may cause bruises and damage the bones that surround and protect the eyes. Blows like this may also rupture the blood vessels of the eye and damage internal eye structures, causing loss of vision. Wounds from sharp objects penetrating the eyeball are serious because of the internal damage they can cause and the infection that can result.

Cover only one eye (the most seriously injured eye) to avoid the psychological stress that the casualty may suffer when both eyes are covered. If both eyes must be covered due to serious injury, (e.g. intense light burn from arc welding), reassure the casualty often by explaining what is being done and why.

First aid for lacerations and bruises around the eye

Lacerated eyelids usually bleed profusely because of their rich blood supply. A dressing on the area will usually control bleeding. Never apply pressure to the eyeball—this may force fluid out of the eyeball and cause permanent damage to the eye.

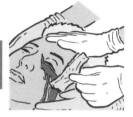 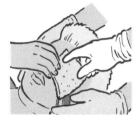 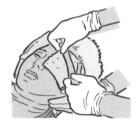

 First aid for an embedded object in or near the eyeball

Give first aid for an embedded object in or near the eyeball as for any embedded object—leave the object where it is, stop the bleeding and get medical help. Prevent the embedded object from moving since movement could cause further damage to the eyeball.

1 Begin ESM—do a scene survey. Lay the casualty down and, if available, have a bystander support the head to reduce movement.

2 Place dressings, preferably sterile, around the embedded object. Place padding or dressings around the object in a "log cabin" fashion, to stabilize the object. Make sure there is no pressure on the eyeball.

3 Arrange transportation of the casualty on a stretcher to medical help as soon as possible.

First aid for an extruded eyeball

When the eyeball has been thrust out of its socket, it is called "extruded."

Do not try to put the eye back into position.

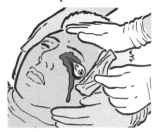

1   Begin ESM—do a scene survey. Lay the casualty down, and if available, have a bystander support the head to reduce movement. Wash your hands or put on gloves.

2   Gently cover the eyeball and socket with a moist dressing. Hold this in place with tape and more dressings.

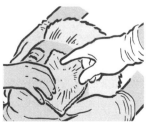

3   Place the casualty face up on a stretcher with the head immobilized for transportation to medical help.

4   Serious injury may result if the casualty is not kept quiet and is not moved carefully by stretcher. Give ongoing casualty care until handover.

Burns

Burns are injuries to the skin and other tissues caused by heat, radiation or chemicals. They are a leading cause of injury in the home. Young children and elderly people are especially at risk of being burned, and at these ages, burn injuries are more serious.

Types of burns

Based on the mechanism of injury, there are four types of burns.

5

Heat burns (also called "thermal" burns)

Burns from too much heat applied to the body are the most familiar kind of burns. Common heat sources include o pen flames, like candles or fire, and hot objects like stoves or car engines. A scald is a heat burn caused by hot liquid or steam. Heat burns can also be caused by friction.

Chemical burns

Chemical burns are often serious because the chemicals continue to burn as long as they remain on the skin. Examples of industrial chemicals that can burn include acids, alkalies, phenols and phosphorus. Chemicals kept in the home that can burn include paint stripper, oven cleaner, drain cleaner and rust remover.

Electrical burns

Electrical burns result from contact with an electric current. Although it is heat that causes these burns, electrical burns are considered separately because of the complications caused by the electricity.

Radiation burns

Most people have experienced a radiation burn in the form of a sunburn, where the sun is the source of radiant energy. Other types of radiant energy that can cause burns include X-rays, arc welder's flash and radiation from radioactive material.

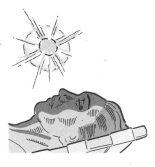

Severity of a burn

The severity of a burn is determined according to the characteristics listed below. Burns are classified as critical, moderate or mild.

5

◆ the depth of the burn—this is called the degree of the burn

◆ the amount of body surface that is burned

◆ the part(s) of the body that is burned

◆ the age and physical condition of the casualty

Burn depth

The skin has two layers, a top layer and a second layer. Underneath the second layer is fat tissue and below that is muscle tissue. The skin protects the body from bacteria, helps control body temperature and keeps body fluid in the body. When the skin is damaged by a burn, it cannot do these functions properly, or at all.

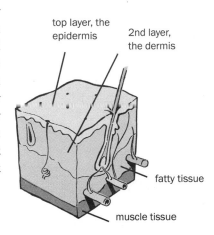

top layer, the epidermis

2nd layer, the dermis

fatty tissue

muscle tissue

The degree of a burn depends on the depth of the tissue damage. The deeper the burn, the more serious it is. In first aid, there are three degrees of burns—first, second and third-degree. Third-degree burns are the most serious.

Estimating the burned area—the rule of nines

A first aider can quickly estimate how much body surface area has been burned using the rule of nines. The body is divided up into areas of either nine or eighteen percent of total body area. Add these areas to quickly calculate the percentage of the body that is affected. The percentages change slightly for a child's body.

5

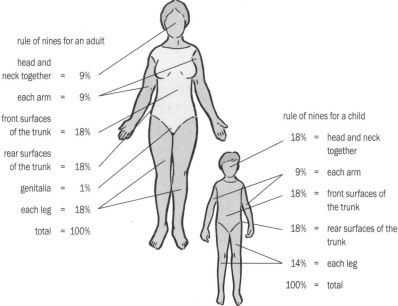

rule of nines for an adult

head and neck together	=	9%
each arm	=	9%
front surfaces of the trunk	=	18%
rear surfaces of the trunk	=	18%
genitalia	=	1%
each leg	=	18%
total	=	100%

rule of nines for a child

18%	=	head and neck together
9%	=	each arm
18%	=	front surfaces of the trunk
18%	=	rear surfaces of the trunk
14%	=	each leg
100%	=	total

Another way to estimate burned area

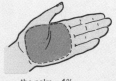

the palm = 1%

The area of the casualty's palm equals one percent of the casualty's body surface area. With this information, you can estimate the percentage of the body that is burned.

Critical, moderate and mild burns

The burns listed below are critical, meaning they may be life-threatening or can cause serious, life-long disability or disfigurement.

◆ any burn that interferes with breathing, including burns to the face and throat and inhalation injuries

◆ any burn where there is also a serious soft tissue injury or fracture

◆ any burn where the skin bends, including the elbows, neck, knees, etc.

◆ all electrical burns

◆ most chemical burns

◆ burns to casualties under two or over fifty years old—these people don't tolerate burns very well

◆ burns to casualties who have serious underlying medical conditions including diabetes, seizure disorders, hypertension, respiratory difficulties, or mental illness

The table on page 210 shows the severity of burns based on the degree of the burn, the percentage of the body burned, and the part of the body burned.

5

Severity of burns			
Percentage of body with burns:			
Severity	3rd degree	2nd degree	1st degree
critical burn	>10% (>2% in a child) or any part of the face, hands, feet or genitals	>30% (>20% in a child)	>70%
moderate burn	2–10% face, hands or feet not burned	15–30% (10–20% in a child)	50–70%
minor burn	<2%	<15% (<10% in a child)	<20% face, hands, feet or genitals **not** burned

5

Complications of burns

Burn injuries often affect much more than just the burned tissue. In critical burns, all the major systems of the body can be affected. For this reason, burn casualties need medical help immediately so the extent of the injuries can be properly assessed. Common complications of burns include:

◆ shock caused by the loss of blood or blood plasma to the surrounding tissues. Shock can be aggravated by the pain of the burn

◆ infection because burned skin isn't a good barrier to bacteria, and the injured area may provide a place for bacteria to breed

◆ breathing problems if the face or throat is burned, or the casualty has inhaled smoke, fumes or steam

◆ swelling because tight clothing and jewellery will cut off circulation when the area swells

Inhalation injuries

Inhalation injuries are often associated with burns. These occur when the casualty breathes steam, smoke or fumes. The signs of an inhalation injury may appear quickly, or may become apparent hours after the incident. For this reason, keep checking the casualty and asking if her breathing is alright. If the casualty begins to cough or wheeze, you should suspect an inhalation injury. The signs, symptoms and first aid for an inhalation injury are given on page 100.

Recognizing burns

5

Use the signs and symptoms of burns to recognize them and determine the degree of the burn (sometimes this is difficult to do). The mechanism of injury will also give you clues as to the severity of the burn and whether the injury is critical.

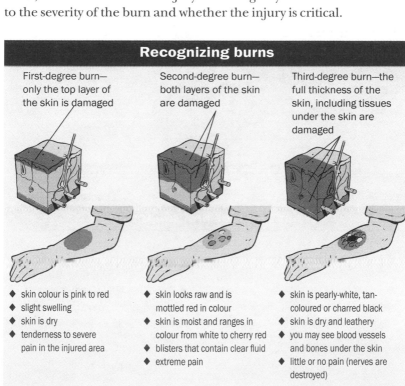

Recognizing burns

First-degree burn—only the top layer of the skin is damaged

Second-degree burn—both layers of the skin are damaged

Third-degree burn—the full thickness of the skin, including tissues under the skin are damaged

- skin colour is pink to red
- slight swelling
- skin is dry
- tenderness to severe pain in the injured area

- skin looks raw and is mottled red in colour
- skin is moist and ranges in colour from white to cherry red
- blisters that contain clear fluid
- extreme pain

- skin is pearly-white, tan-coloured or charred black
- skin is dry and leathery
- you may see blood vessels and bones under the skin
- little or no pain (nerves are destroyed)

First aid for heat burns

1 Begin ESM—do the scene survey. Do a primary survey.

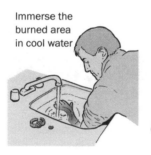

2 Cool the burn right away—immerse it in cool water. If you can't do this, pour cool water on the area or cover it with a clean, wet cloth.

Cool the burn until the pain has lessened. This will reduce the temperature of the burned area, and reduce tissue damage, swelling, blistering and relieve the pain.

5

Immerse the burned area in cool water

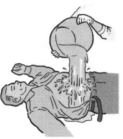

Pour cool water on the burn

Cover the burned area with cloths soaked with cool water

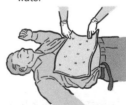

Precautions for first aid for burns

◆ Do not breathe on, cough over or touch the burned area.

◆ Do not break blisters.

◆ Do not remove clothing that is stuck to the burned area.

◆ Do not use butter, lotions*, ointments* or oily dressings on a burn.

◆ Do not cover a burn with cotton wool or other fluffy material.

◆ Do not use adhesive dressings.

◆ Do not cool the casualty too much. Once the area is cooled, take action to keep the casualty warm.

* Sunburn lotions and ointments can be used on minor sunburn.

3 Loosen or remove anything on the burned area that is tight—this means   jewellery and tight clothing. Do this as soon as you can, before the injury swells. Don't remove anything that is stuck.

4 When the pain has lessened, loosely cover the burn with a clean, lint-free dressing. If the area is large, use a sheet. Secure the dressing with tape, making sure there is no tape on the burned area.

5 Give ongoing casualty care including arranging for medical help, first aid for shock and monitoring the casualty.

5

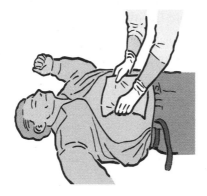

Burn dressings

A good burn dressing is sterile, lint-free and won't stick to the injury when it is removed. If you don't have something like this, use something clean and lint-free, like a linen sheet.

Another type of burn dressing is the "gelled water" burn dressing, e.g. Water-Jel®. These sterile dressings are coated with a jelly-like substance that is mostly water. As such, the dressings are effective in cooling the burn, keeping it clean and providing pain relief. Use these dressings according to the instructions on the package.

First aid for chemical burns

A corrosive chemical will keep burning as long as it is on the skin. The faster you get the chemical off the skin, the less tissue damage there will be.

1   Begin ESM—do a scene survey. Do a primary survey.

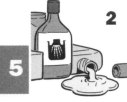

2   Remove the chemical from the body by flushing the area with large amounts of cool water. Don't delay flushing to remove clothing. Remove the clothing while flushing. If the chemical is a dry powder, quickly brush off any loose chemical with a cloth before flushing.

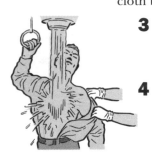

3   Continue flushing the area with water for 15 to 20 minutes.

4   When the area has been flushed, loosely cover the burn with a clean, lint-free, preferably sterile dressing. If the area is large, use a sheet. Secure the dressing with tape, making sure no tape touches the burned area.

5   Give ongoing casualty care including arranging for medical help. If the casualty complains that the burning sensation increases, flush the area again for at least 10 minutes.

Using chemical neutralizers

Do not use chemical neutralizers such as vinegar, soda or alcohol, to treat any chemical burn, unless advised to do so by a medical doctor.

If you work with chemicals, make sure you know the specific first aid for the chemicals in your workplace. The MSDS* for each chemical contains this information.

* *material safety data sheet—see page 393*

First aid for chemical burns to the eye

The eyes can be permanently injured by corrosive c hemicals in either solid or liquid form. Casualties normally suffer intense pain and are very sensitive to light. Give first aid as follows:

1   Begin ESM—do a scene survey. If you can, put gloves on or wash your hands.

2   Sit or lay the casualty down. Tilt the head back and turn it slightly to the injured side. If only one eye is injured, protect the uninjured eye.

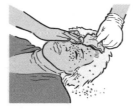

3   If the chemical is a dry powder, brush away whatever is on the skin. Use a cloth to brush the powder away from the face. Do not use your bare hands.

4   Flush the injured eye with cool water. Since pain may make it hard for the casualty to keep the eye open, gently open the eye with your fingers. Flush the eye for at least 15 minutes.

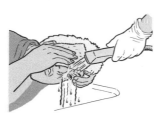
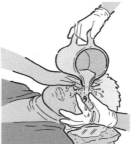

5   Cover the injured eye with dressings. If both eyes are injured, cover the more seriously injured eye. Only cover both eyes if the casualty is more comfortable that way. Covering both eyes, so the casualty can't see, adds to the stress of the scene. If you do cover both eyes, reassure the casualty by explaining what is being done and why.

6   Get medical help right away and give ongoing casualty care.

5

If the casualty is wearing contact lenses

Don't waste time trying to remove contact lenses. Flush the eyes for 15 minutes—this may wash the lenses out. If not, have the casualty remove them. Lenses exposed to chemicals should be thrown away (so it doesn't matter if they are washed away during flushing).

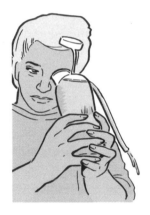

When there is a risk of eye injury from chemicals, proper eye-wash equipment should be kept nearby.

 First aid for electrical burns

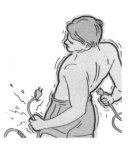
An electrical burn may be more serious than it appears. An electrical current going through the body can cause breathing to stop and/or the heart to stop. Also, an electric shock can violently throw the casualty. Head/spinal injuries, fractures or dislocations may be present. There is also the danger of electrical injury to the first aider.

1 Begin ESM—do a scene survey. Make sure there is no further danger from electricity. If you are not sure, don't put yourself in danger—call the power company or other officials to make the scene safe. Only turn electricity off at the source—never try to cut or move live wires. If high voltages are involved, all you can do is keep others out of the area until the power is shut off.

Examine the scene carefully. Does it look like the casualty was thrown? If so, suspect a head or spinal injury.

2 Do a primary survey and give first aid for life-threatening injuries.

3 Do a secondary survey to locate burns and any fractures, dislocations, etc. Look for both entry and exit burns.

5

Two kinds of electrical burns

Electrical burns can be either flash burns or contact burns. Although you may not be able to tell the type of burn at an emergency scene, knowing the two types helps to understand electrical burn injuries.

A flash burn results when electricity arcs (jumps) from the electric source to the casualty. When electricity arcs, it produces intense heat for a very short time. This heat causes flash burn, which can be a very deep third-degree burn. In some cases the tissue is completely burned away, leaving a hole.

The electricity does not travel through the body in flash burn, so tissue damage inside the body is usually not severe.

In a contact burn, electricity travels through the body. Here, the body conducts the electricity from one place to another, and the electricity travels along a path through the body. The body may be burned at both the point where the electricity entered the body and where it exited. There may also be severe tissue damage inside the body, along the path the electricity followed.

4 Give first aid for the entry and exit burns by covering them with clean, dry dressings. Tape these in place, making sure the tape doesn't touch damaged skin.

5 Give first aid for any fractures or dislocations—see Chapter 6.

6 Give ongoing casualty care including getting medical help, giving first aid for shock and monitoring the casualty.

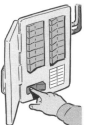

Shut off power at the source before entering the scene

When power lines are down

◆ Inspect the emergency scene as you arrive. If there is a possibility of a downed power line or a weakened pole, go no further. Don't leave your vehicle until you have inspected the surrounding area, looking for downed power lines.

◆ Stay inside your vehicle if it is touching power lines. Wait for authorities to arrive, than follow their instructions.

◆ If you suspect or see any downed power lines, don't let anyone enter the area. When you are sure no one will enter the area, notify the power company.

◆ With high voltages, electricity can travel through the ground, energizing the area around the power lines. If the soles of your feet tingle as you enter an area, you've gone too far—get back.

◆ Assume all downed power lines are live unless the power company crew says otherwise. A high voltage wire may be unpredictable—it may jump to an object for a better ground. Stay well away from any wires.

◆ Remember that vehicles, guardrails, metal fences, etc., conduct electricity.

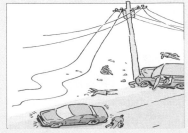

First aid for radiation burns

Radiation burns are caused by radiant energy—energy that radiates from a source. Sunburn and snowblindness are radiation burns caused by sunlight. Sunlamps at tanning parlours can also cause radiation burns to the skin and eyes. Other causes of radiation burns include X-rays and the flash of arc welding.

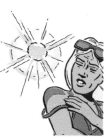

 First aid for sunburn

Sunburns can range in severity from those that are mildly uncomfortable to those that are serious, cover a large portion of the body, and are complicated by heatstroke. For minor sunburn, give first aid as follows:

1 Begin ESM—do a scene survey and a primary survey. Get out of the sun. Gently sponge the area with cool water or cover with a wet towel, to relieve the pain. Repeat this step as needed to relieve pain.

2 Pat the skin dry and put on a medicated sunburn ointment or lotion (these can cause an allergic reaction in some people). Apply the lotion according to directions on the package.

3 Protect burned areas from further exposure to the sun.

4 Don't break any blisters—doing so may promote infection. If large areas of the skin begin to blister, get medical help.

5 If the casualty begins to vomit, or develops a fever, give first aid for heatstroke (see page 311) and get medical help.

First aid for burns from X-rays and nuclear radiation

There is no specific first aid for radiation burns from X-rays or radioactive material. Give first aid following the guidelines for first aid for heat burns. In an environment where there is radioactive material, protect yourself accordingly.

First aid for intense light burns to the eye(s)

5

Burns to the eyes may be caused by intense light such as direct or reflected sunlight and arc welder's flash. Snowblindness is a common injury of this kind. As with a sunburn, the casualty may not feel the tissue damage happening but will develop symptoms several hours after exposure. Signs and symptoms include:

◆ sensitivity to light

◆ pain

◆ a gritty feeling in the eyes

Give first aid as follows:

1 Begin ESM—do a scene survey and a primary survey. Wash your hands or put on gloves.

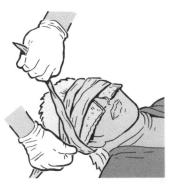

2 Cover the eyes to cool them and keep the light out. The casualty will be temporarily blinded, so reassure her often and explain what you are doing. If the casualty doesn't want both eyes covered, even after an explanation and reassurance, cover only one eye.

3 Get medical help and give ongoing casualty care.

How to put out a fire on your clothes

If your clothing catches fire:

1 **Stop** – moving

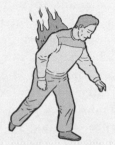

2 **Drop** – to the ground

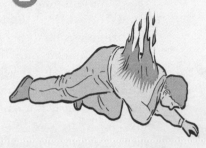

3 **and roll** – several times to put flames out

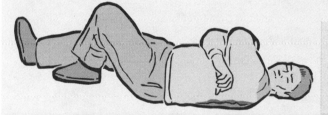

 Don't run

This only fans the flames.

How to exit a smoke-filled room

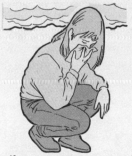

If you can, cover your mouth and nose with a wet cloth

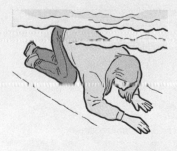

Hot smoke rises—keep your head low as you crawl under the smoke

Bites and stings

Animal and human bites

Animal and human bites that cause puncture wounds or lacerations may carry contaminated saliva into the body. Human bites and the bites of domestic animals are dangerous because of the risk of infection. The most common human bites in adults are to the hand and knuckles. Bites from wild animals, such as bats, foxes, skunks and raccoons, may carry the rabies virus which could be fatal if the casualty does not get medical help quickly. To be safe, always give first aid for an animal bite as if the animal had rabies, until it is proved otherwise. Any bite that breaks the skin is serious.

More about rabies

Rabies is an acute viral disease of the nervous system that is always fatal if not treated. Rabies should be suspected in domestic animals if they behave in an unusual way (the gentle dog or cat that attacks for no apparent reason and shows no fear of its owner) and in all attacks by wild animals. The rabies virus can be transmitted to anyone who handles a diseased animal or who touches the area of the wound that carries the virus.

Be especially careful when giving first aid to anyone you suspect may have been exposed to rabies and in handling the live or dead animal involved. Wear gloves and/or scrub your hands thoroughly after contact to reduce the risk of infection.

If the animal can be captured without risk to you or others, it should be kept for examination. If the animal must be killed, try to keep the head intact so that the brain can be examined for the rabies virus.

Even if a person has been exposed to a rabid animal, full-blown rabies can be prevented if immunization against the disease is given quickly.

First aid for animal/human bites

1   Start ESM—do a scene survey. Protect yourself by wearing gloves when giving first aid or handling an animal that may be infected.

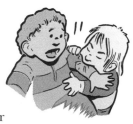

2   Do a primary survey and give first aid for any life-threatening conditions.

3   Examine the wound to see if the skin was broken.

4   If there is bleeding, allow moderate bleeding of the wound—this helps to cleanse the wound.

5

5   Wash the wound with an antiseptic soap or detergent. Apply a dressing and bandage.

6   If the skin was broken, get medical help as soon as possible.

All animal and human bites that break the skin should be seen by a doctor.

Snakebite

Rattlesnakes are the only poisonous snakes found in the wild in Canada. Varieties of this snake are found in parts of British Columbia, Alberta, Saskatchewan and Ontario but they are not numerous, and snakebites are not common. If you are travelling to areas where there are other poisonous snakes, learn the first aid for snakebites in that area.

A rattlesnake's bite leaves one or two puncture holes in the skin. Venom is usually, but not always, injected into the casualty. If it is, the casualty will feel a burning sensation. This is followed by swelling and discoloration, severe pain, weakness, sweating, nausea, vomiting and chills. Breathing may be affected.

First aid for snakebite

1   Begin ESM—do a scene survey. Make sure there is no danger of a second snakebite to either the casualty or yourself.

2   Do a primary survey.

3   Place the casualty at rest in a semi-sitting position and keep the affected limb below heart level. By placing the casualty at rest, the venom won't spread as quickly.

4   Flush the bite with soapy water, if available. Do not apply cold compresses or ice. Apply a pressure immobilization bandage around the entire length of the bitten extremity. This is an effective and safe way to slow circulation of the venom.

5   Immobilize the limb as for a fracture (see chapter 6).

6   Give ongoing casualty care and transport the casualty to medical help as soon as possible.

Precautions when dealing with snakes and snakebite

◆ most snakes will be within 10 metres of the place where the bite took place—be careful

◆ do not let a snakebite casualty walk if there is any other method of transportation to medical help

◆ do not give the casualty alcoholic beverages

◆ do not cut the puncture marks or try to suck poison out with your mouth

◆ do not apply ice—this could cause more damage

◆ if the snake is killed, bring it to medical help for identification, but do not touch the snake directly. Avoid the snake's head—a dead snake still may have a bite reflex

Insect bites and stings

In most people, an insect bite or sting causes only a painful swelling with redness and itching at the site of the sting. But some people are severely allergic to these stings and being stung may cause a life-threatening allergic reaction.

Ask the casualty if he has ever had an allergic reaction to a sting before. Also look for the signs of an allergic reaction. If you suspect the casualty is having an allergic reaction to a sting, place him at rest and give first aid for a severe allergic reaction (see page 107).

5

Signs and symptoms at the site of a bite or sting

◆ sudden pain

◆ swelling

◆ heat

◆ redness

◆ itching

Signs and symptoms of an allergic reaction to a bite or sting

◆ general itching, rash

◆ a bump on the skin that may be white, pink, reddish or blotchy

◆ generalized swelling—especially of the airway

◆ weakness, headache

◆ fever

◆ breathing difficulties that may be severe

◆ anxiety, abdominal cramps, vomiting

First aid for an insect bite or sting

1   Begin ESM—do a scene survey. Do a primary survey and give first aid for the ABCs. Examine the sting site closely, looking for the stinger that may still be in the skin.

If it is there, remove it by carefully scraping it and the attached poison sac from the skin. Use the sharp edge like a knife blade or a credit card. Don't use tweezers, fingers or anything that may squeeze more poison into the body.

2   For the irritation at the site of the sting, apply rubbing alcohol or a paste of baking soda and water. Ice can also be used. Don't use alcohol near the eyes.

3   For serious reactions that affect breathing or cause swelling of the airway, assist the casualty to take their own medication (autoinjector). For more information on how to use an auto-injector, see page 108.

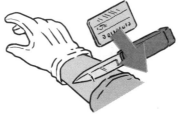

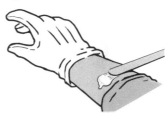

If the sting is in the mouth, give the person a mouthwash of one teaspoonful of baking soda in a glass of water, or a piece of ice to suck on. If there is swelling in the mouth, or if there is difficulty breathing, monitor the person closely and get medical help.

5

Ticks

Ticks are found in abundance throughout the forests in some parts of Canada. They drop from the foliage onto animals and humans, biting through the skin and anchoring themselves to the tissue with barbed mouth parts. A tick will suck the host's (the person or animal) blood for many hours and may become quite large. At the end of the meal, the tick detaches itself and drops off.

Poison from the tick may be harmful. They sometimes carry disease that can be transmitted to humans. A tick on the body should be removed. If one tick is found, check your body and clothing thoroughly for others.

5

First aid for bites from ticks

1   Begin ESM—do a scene survey. Remove the embedded tick. Grasp it as close to the casualty's skin as possible and pull away from the skin with even, steady pressure. Avoid squashing an engorged tick. Infected blood may spurt into your eyes, mouth, or a cut on the surface of your skin. If you don't have tweezers, wear gloves or cover your hand with a plastic bag or tissue paper. If the tick is full of blood, wear eye protection.

2   Keep the dislodged tick and bring it to medical help for identification.

3   Clean the area with soap and water and apply an antiseptic to prevent infection. Wash your hands.

Ticks can carry various diseases which may cause symptoms several days after exposure. If the site of the bite shows any sign of infection, or there are other worrisome signs or symptoms within the next week, get medical help.

Leeches

Leeches live in swamps, ponds, lakes and stagnant water. Some feed on the warm blood of animals or humans. A leech makes a tiny cut in the skin, which may not be felt at the time, and attaches itself to feed on blood. Once a leech is attached, trying to pull it off often doesn't work— the leech may tear into smaller parts, making it even harder to remove those parts still attached. This may increase the risk of infection.

5

 ### First aid for lesions from leeches

1 Begin ESM—do a scene survey.

2 Detach the leech by first using a fingernail to push the head end of the leech off of the skin.

It is important to note that the head end is the smaller, skinnier part of the leech–not the larger end. After the head is released, use a fingernail to push the larger end off.

3 Once the leech is removed there will be some bleeding due to the anticoagulant produced by the leech. Clean the area with water and apply a paste of baking soda and water. This will also relieve irritation.

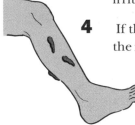

4 If the site of the bite shows any sign of infection in the next week, the casualty should get medical help.

Jellyfish

Worldwide, there are about 2,000 different species of jellyfish. In Atlantic Canada, the Arctic Red jellyfish and White Moon jellyfish are the more common species. In the Pacific region, the more common jellyfish are the Fried Egg, Moon, Water, Arctic Red, and By-The-Wind Sailor. Jellyfish can be found in any body of water, whether salt water or fresh. Jellyfish that are found in Canada may "sting" a person out of fear or protection from a predator.

Jellyfish that have been known to cause death are located in tropical climates and have not been located near Canada.

All jellyfish sting their prey using nematocysts, which in simple terms are "stingers". These stingers may contain venom which can be harmful, but more commonly cause an unpleasant stinging or burning sensation.

 First aid for jellyfish stings

1   Begin ESM—do a scene survey. Ensure casualty is out of the water.

2   Ensure safety—wear gloves and avoid touching the affected part.

3   Apply as much vinegar as possible to the affected area. Vinegar will stop the stingers from releasing venom.

4   To help relieve pain, bathe the affected part in warm water, as warm as the casualty can tolerate for about 20 minutes.

5   Do not apply cold water. Cold water helps the stingers to continue releasing any venom.

6   If signs of infection occur, seek medical help.

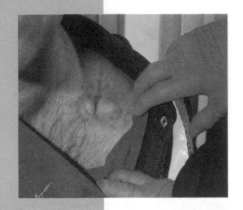

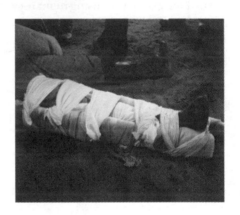

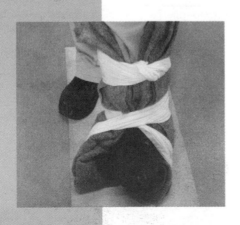

CHAPTER **6**

Injuries to Bones and Joints

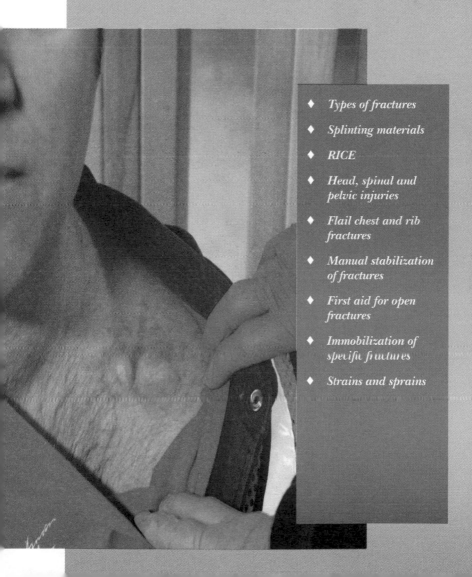

- ♦ *Types of fractures*
- ♦ *Splinting materials*
- ♦ *RICE*
- ♦ *Head, spinal and pelvic injuries*
- ♦ *Flail chest and rib fractures*
- ♦ *Manual stabilization of fractures*
- ♦ *First aid for open fractures*
- ♦ *Immobilization of specific fractures*
- ♦ *Strains and sprains*

Introduction

Injuries to bones, joints and muscles can range from minor to very severe. These injuries are common and, as a first aider, you will likely encounter them. Although injuries to bones, joints and muscles are usually not life-threatening, they can be painful, debilitating, and can cause life-long aggravation, disability and deformity. Appropriate first aid for these injuries can make the injury more bearable for the casualty and reduce the chances of lifelong effects from the injury.

This chapter describes different types of bone, joint and muscle injuries and the appropriate first aid. The functions of bones, joints and muscles are described in Appendix C, The Body and How it Works.

6

Injuries to bones

Bones break, and broken bones are your concern as a first aider. A break or crack in a bone is called a fracture. A fracture is either closed or open:

◆ a **closed fracture** is where the skin over the fracture is not broken

◆ an **open fracture** is where the skin over the fracture is broken—this could cause serious infection, even if the wound is very small

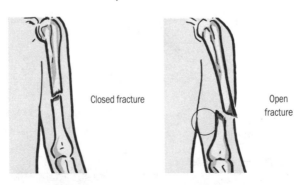

Closed fracture

Open fracture

Other terms are used to describe particular types of fractures—some of these are shown below. The first aider often cannot determine the type of fracture that has occurred.

Types of fractures

depression fracture—skull is fractured inward

complicated fracture—broken bone has caused damage to internal organs

transverse fracture—bone is broken straight across

6

spiral fracture—bone is broken by twisting

oblique fracture—bone is broken on a steep angle

greenstick fracture—bone is not broken right through

Mechanism of injury

A **fracture** can be caused by a direct force (e.g. a punch or kick), an indirect force (e.g. a fall), or by a twisting force. Certain bone diseases, such as osteoporosis, make bones very brittle and they can break without much force.

Signs and symptoms of a fracture

One or more of the following signs and symptoms will be present when a bone is fractured:

◆ pain and tenderness—it is worse when the injury is touched or moved

◆ loss of function—the casualty cannot use the injured part

◆ a wound—the bone ends may be sticking out

◆ deformity—any unnatural shape or unnatural position of a bone or joint

◆ unnatural movement

6

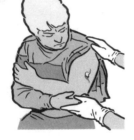

◆ shock—this increases with the severity of the injury

◆ crepitus—a grating sensation or sound that can often be felt or heard when the broken ends of bone rub together (don't test for this)

◆ swelling and bruising—fluid accumulates in the tissues around the fracture

Injuries to joints

A **joint** is located where two or more bones come together. Joints may be injured when the bones and surrounding tissues are forced to move beyond their normal range. When a joint is forced to move more than it should, the following can happen:

◆ the bones may break, resulting in a fracture

◆ the ligaments may stretch and tear, resulting in a sprain

◆ the bone ends may move out of proper position
  resulting in a dislocation

Sprains

A **sprain** is an injury to a ligament and can range from
a stretched to a completely torn ligament. Without
specialized training it is difficult to determine the degree
of a sprain—be cautious and give first aid as if the injury
is serious. Sprains of the wrist, ankle, knee and shoulder
are most common.

The signs and symptoms of sprains may include:

◆ pain that may be severe and increase with movement
  of the joint

◆ loss of function

◆ swelling and discoloration

6

Dislocations

When the bone surfaces that come together at a joint are
no longer in proper contact, the joint is said to be
dislocated. A **dislocation** stretches and tears the
fibrous capsule that holds the joint together.

A dislocation can be caused by a severe twist of a joint
or by indirect force. The joints most frequently
dislocated are the shoulder, elbow, thumb, finger, lower
jaw and knee. A dislocated bone can put pressure on
nearby blood vessels and impair or cut off circulation
below the injury—this is a serious complication of
dislocation that the first aider should look for.

Signs and symptoms of a dislocation

The signs and symptoms of a dislocation are similar to those of a fracture, and may include:

◆ deformity or abnormal appearance, a dislocated shoulder may make the arm look longer

◆ pain and tenderness aggravated by movement

◆ loss of normal function; the joint may be "locked" in one position

◆ swelling of the joint

6

 ### General first aid for injuries to bones and joints

Below is general first aid for injuries to bones and joints. The methods of immobilizing different bones and joints follow this general approach.

The aims of first aid for bone and joint injuries are to prevent further tissue damage and to reduce pain.

1   Begin ESM—do a scene survey. Assess the mechanism of injury. If you suspect a head or spinal injury, call for medical help, then steady and support the head before continuing.

2   Do a primary survey and give first aid for life-threatening injuries.

3   Steady and support any obvious fractures or dislocations found in the primary survey (during the rapid body check). Dress any obvious wounds to prevent further contamination. Protect any protruding bones.

4 Do a secondary survey to the extent needed. When you find a bone or joint injury, carefully and gently expose the injured area. You may have to cut clothing to do this without moving the injured part. Take a good look at the entire injured area to determine the extent of the injury. Look for a wound indicating an open fracture. Most open fractures have only a small wound, but there is still danger of serious infection.

Check the circulation below the injury. If circulation is impaired, medical help is needed urgently.

5 Steady and support the injured part—you can do this, a bystander can do this, or the casualty may be able to do this. Maintain support until medical help takes over, or the injury is immobilized.

6 Now decide what action is best. If medical help is on the way and will arrive soon, steady and support the injury with your hands until they arrive. If medical help will be delayed, or if the casualty needs to be transported, immobilize the injury. Consider the following when making your decision.

Are there other risks to the casualty? Are there risks to yourself or others?

If medical help can get to the scene, how long will it take?

Do you have the materials needed to properly immobilize the injury?

How long will it take to immobilize the injury compared to how long it will take for medical help to arrive?

Use RICE for injuries to bones, joints and muscles

Most injuries to bones, joints and muscles benefit from **RICE**, which stands for:

◆ Rest

◆ Immobilize

◆ Cold

◆ Elevation

Rest means stopping the activity that caused the injury and staying off it until a doctor tells you it's O.K. For a minor injury, gentle use of the injured part is okay provided you can easily tolerate the pain.

6

Immobilize means suspecting a fracture whenever there is an injury to an arm or a leg and taking steps to prevent movement of the injured limb. Immobilization may mean using a sling for a shoulder joint injury or a splint to immobilize the joint above and the joint below the injury.

Cold means applying cold to the injury as soon as you can once the injury has been immobilized. The cold narrows the blood vessels, reducing pain, swelling and bruising. Use a commercial cold pack, an improvised ice pack or a cold compress (see page 239) for more about using cold.

Apply cold over the entire injured area—15 minutes on, 15 minutes off.

Elevation means raising the injured part if possible. Only elevate if it will not cause more pain or harm to the casualty. Elevation helps to reduce swelling and makes it easier for fluids to drain away from the injury. This in turn, helps reduce swelling (don't elevate a "locked" joint).

When to use RICE

Use RICE while waiting for medical help to arrive or while transporting a casualty to medical help. Even the most minor injuries will benefit from RICE.

ICE warnings

◆ Do not put an ice bag directly on the skin; always have a layer of cloth between the ice and the skin.

◆ Do not use cold when there is an open wound or if the skin is "tented" or pushed up from underneath by an injured bone.

◆ Do not use ice if the casualty is sensitive to the cold—ask the casualty if she is sensitive to cold and check for a skin reaction, such as a rash or blisters.

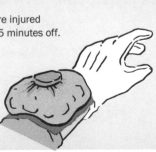

When and how to use cold on injuries

Applying cold to an injury is generally good first aid and you should do it as soon as possible following the guidelines below.

Use cold:

◆ as soon as possible after an injury has taken place

◆ when pain, swelling and bruising are the dominant factors, as in strains, sprains, bruises, dislocations, or when muscle spasm is present e.g. a "charley horse"

◆ for up to 48 hours after injury

Do not use cold:

◆ on an open injury

◆ if circulation below the injury is impaired or the casualty has known circulatory disorders

◆ if the skin at the injury site is "tented" by pressure from broken bones under the skin

◆ if the casualty is unconscious or semi-conscious, since she cannot tell you if discomfort or frostbite occurs

◆ if the casualty is sensitive to cold (ask the casualty about this) or if the cold causes hives to appear.

Different ways to apply cold

Use a cold compress. Soak a towel in cold water, wring out the excess water and wrap the towel around the injured part.

Use an ice bag. Make one by filling a rubber or plastic bag two-thirds full of crushed ice, forcing out any excess air from the bag, and sealing the opening to make it watertight. A bag of frozen vegetables, like peas or corn, works well. Wrap the bag in a towel and apply it carefully to the injured part. Replace the ice as necessary.

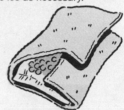

To use a commercial cold pack, follow the manufacturer's directions to activate the chemicals that make it cold. Wrap the cold pack in a towel before applying it to the injured area. Caution must be used, as these sometimes leak.

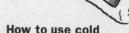

How to use cold

Put the cold compress, ice bag or cold pack on the injured area (with a cloth between the skin and the ice bag or cold pack). Leave the cold in place for 15 minutes. Then take the cold off for 15 minutes. This will help to avoid the casualty suffering frostbite. Repeat this 15-minutes-on 15-minutes-off cycle for the first 48 hours following the injury. Always be alert for signs of frostbite.

6

7 Apply cold to the injury, as appropriate, and elevate the injured part (see RICE, on page 238).

8 Give ongoing casualty care until medical help arrives. Monitor circulation below the injury site.

Head injuries

A "head injury" refers to a serious injury of the head where brain function is, or may be, affected. Head injuries include skull fractures, brain concussion and brain compression. Such injuries are frequently complicated by unconsciousness. Fractures at the base of the skull often involve injury to the cervical spine. For this reason, when you suspect a head injury, you should also suspect a neck injury.

6

Signs and symptoms of head injuries

The following signs and symptoms indicate a possible fracture of the skull or facial bones, concussion or compression:

- deformed skull
- swollen, bruised or bleeding scalp
- straw-coloured fluid or blood coming from the nose or ear(s)
- bruising around the eyes (black eye) or behind the ears
- nausea, vomiting, especially in children

- confused, dazed, possibly combative
- semi-conscious or unconscious
- stopped breathing or irregular respiration
- very slow pulse rate
- pupils are of unequal size
- pain at the injury site
- weakened or paralysed arms and/or legs

◆ pain when swallowing or moving the jaw

◆ wounds in the mouth

◆ knocked-out teeth

◆ shock

◆ convulsions

Skull fracture

Fractures of the skull may be the result of direct force or an indirect force that is transmitted through the bones. Fractures may occur in the cranium, at the base of the skull, or in the face. Facial fractures include the nose, the bones around the eyes, the upper jaw and the lower jaw. Fractures of the jaw are often complicated by wounds inside the mouth.

6

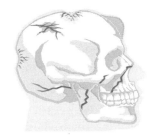

An unconscious casualty with a head injury may vomit. Be ready to turn the casualty to the side (as a unit if possible) and clear the airway quickly.

Helmets

Helmets are designed to protect the wearer from fractures. They are not actually designed to protect against concussion or compression injury. If you see signs or symptoms of this type of injury, get help immediately.

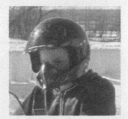

First aid for head injury, including fracture of the skull

First aid for fractures of the skull depends on the fracture site and the signs. Whenever there is a skull fracture, a spinal injury should be suspected—give first aid as if there was a fractured neck. The head and neck should be immobilized accordingly.

1   Begin ESM—start the scene survey. When you recognize that there may be a head injury, tell the casualty not to move and get medical help. Steady and support the head with your hands as soon as possible. Assess responsiveness.

2   Perform a primary survey. If there is no breathing, begin CPR with 30 compressions (see Chapter 4). After the initial 30 compressions, open the airway using the head-tilt chin lift. This is necessary to establish an airway, regardless of movement of the spine.

3   If blood or fluid is coming from the ear canal, secure a sterile dressing lightly over the ear, making sure fluids can drain.

4   Protect areas of depression, lumps, bumps, or scalp wounds where an underlying skull fracture is suspected. Use thick, compressible, soft dressings bandaged in place. Avoid pressure on the fracture site.

5   Warn the casualty not to blow her nose if there is blood or fluid coming from it. Do not restrict blood flow. Wipe away any trickling blood to prevent it from entering the mouth, causing breathing difficulties.

6   Give ongoing casualty care until medical help takes over (see page 60).

First aid for fractures of the facial bones and jaw

If the bones of the face or jaw are broken, assess the mechanism of injury for a head or spinal injury.

1   Begin ESM—start the scene survey. If you suspect a head injury, tell the casualty not to move and get medical help. Steady and support the head with your hands as soon as possible.

2   Do a primary survey. Check the airway and make sure there is nothing in the mouth. Remove any knocked-out teeth or loose dentures and maintain drainage for blood and saliva.

3   Position the casualty. If there is no suspected head or spinal injury:

◆ place the conscious casualty in a sitting position with head well forward to allow any fluids to drain freely

◆ if the casualty cannot sit comfortably, place her in the recovery position

◆ place the unconscious breathing casualty in the recovery position. If the casualty vomits, support the jaw with the palm of your hand and turn the head to the uninjured side

If there is a suspected head or spinal injury, steady and support the casualty in the position found until medical help takes over (see page 249)

4   Get medical help and give ongoing casualty care. Check the casualty's level of consciousness and airway often.

If transporting the casualty on a stretcher, ensure good drainage from the mouth and nose so that breathing will not be impaired.

Concussion and compression

Concussion is a temporary disturbance of brain function usually caused by a blow to the head or neck. The casualty may become unconscious but usually for only a few moments. The casualty may say he "sees stars." Common causes of concussion include traffic collisions, falls and sports injuries. The casualty usually recovers quickly, but there is a chance of serious brain injury. Use both the mechanism of injury and the signs and symptoms below to assess for concussion or compression.

Signs and symptoms of concussion

◆ partial or complete loss of consciousness, usually of short duration

◆ shallow breathing

◆ nausea and vomiting when regaining consciousness

◆ casualty says she is (or was) "seeing stars"

◆ loss of memory of events immediately preceding and following the injury

◆ severe overall headache (not local scalp pain)

Compression is a condition of excess pressure on some part of the brain. It may be caused by a buildup of fluids inside the skull, or by a depressed skull fracture where the broken bones are putting pressure on the brain. For example, if a blow to the head causes bleeding in the brain, and the blood cannot drain, it builds up and puts pressure on the brain. This may happen immediately after a blow to the head, or it may take a few hours, days or even weeks for the signs of compression to show. It is very important to monitor a casualty's vital signs and look for other symptoms after a blow to the head.

Shaken Baby Syndrome

Shaken Baby Syndrome (SBS) is a term used to describe the group of signs and symptoms resulting from violent shaking of the head of an infant or small child.

Signs and Symptoms

There are various signs and symptoms of Shaken Baby Syndrome and if the incident is severe, it can lead to severe disability or death. If you suspect a child has been shaken, seek medical attention immediately.

Symptoms include:

◆ lethargy / decreased muscle tone
◆ extreme irritability
◆ decreased appetite, poor feeding or vomiting for no apparent reason
◆ grab-type bruises on arms or chest are rare
◆ no smiling or vocalization
◆ poor sucking or swallowing
◆ rigidity or posturing
◆ difficulty breathing
◆ seizures
◆ head or forehead appears larger than usual or soft-spot on head appears to be bulging
◆ inability to lift head
◆ inability of eyes to focus or track movement or unequal size of pupils

Physical consequences of shaking

When an infant is shaken the brain rotates within the skull cavity, injuring or destroying brain tissue. When shaking occurs, blood vessels feeding the brain can be torn, leading to bleeding around the brain. Blood pools within the skull, sometimes creating more pressure within the skull and possibly causing additional brain damage. Retinal (back of the eye) bleeding is very common.

6

Immediate Consequences

◆ breathing may stop or be compromised

◆ extreme irritability

◆ seizures

◆ limp arms and legs or rigidity/posturing

◆ decreased level of consciousness

◆ vomiting; poor feeding

◆ inability to suck or swallow

◆ heart may stop

◆ death

Long-term consequences may include:

◆ learning disabilities

◆ physical disabilities

◆ visual disabilities or blindness

◆ hearing impairment

◆ speech disabilities

◆ cerebral palsy

◆ seizures

◆ behavior disorders

◆ cognitive impairment

◆ death

Babies' heads are relatively large and heavy, making up about 25% of their total body weight. Their neck muscles are too weak to support such a disproportionately large head.

Babies' brains are immature and more easily injured by shaking.

Babies' blood vessels around the brain are more susceptible to tearing than older children or adults

When:

Often, perpetrators shake an infant or child out of frustration or anger. This most often occurs when the baby won't stop crying. Other triggering events include toilet training difficulties and feeding problems.

For more information on Shaken Baby Syndrome

Contact the National Centre on Shaken Baby Syndrome
1433 North Highway 89

Suite 110

Farmington, UT 84025

801-627-3399

Email: mail@dontshake.org   www.dontshake.org

Signs of compression

The signs of compression are progressive—they usually get worse as time goes on, as more and more pressure is put on the brain.

◆ loss of consciousness

◆ decreasing level of consciousness

◆ nausea and vomiting

◆ unequal size of pupils

◆ one or both pupils don't respond to light

Ongoing casualty care for head injury

6

When a casualty has received a blow to the head or neck that causes unconsciousness or semi-consciousness, immediately suspect a neck injury. Tell the casualty not to move, steady and support the head, and take precautions for a neck injury.

A casualty with a concussion may appear to recover quickly, but there is always the threat of serious injury. Check the casualty for signs of compression. Tell the casualty to get medical help right away for a full evaluation of the injury.

If the casualty is unconscious and you must leave her alone, place her in the recovery position, carefully supporting the head and neck during any movement. If the casualty is face up, monitor breathing continuously. If necessary hold the airway open using the head tilt-chin lift method (or if trained use the jaw-thrust without head-tilt). Send for medical help and give ongoing casualty care.

Any casualty who shows signs of compression following a blow to the head, even after many days, needs medical help immediately.

Spinal injuries

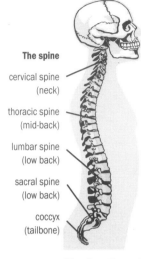

The spine

cervical spine
(neck)

thoracic spine
(mid-back)

lumbar spine
(low back)

sacral spine
(low back)

coccyx
(tailbone)

The spine may be injured anywhere along its length, from the base of the skull to the coccyx. Injury to the spine threatens the spinal cord that runs through it and the nerves that branch out from the cord. Damage to the spinal cord or nerves can result in complete and permanent loss of feeling and paralysis below the point of injury. Injury to the spinal cord at the lower spine may affect only the legs. Damage to the spinal cord in the neck could result in paralysis of the muscles that help control chest movement in breathing. In every emergency situation, assess the possibility of a spinal injury. If it exists at all, give first aid for a spinal injury and get medical help as soon as possible.

Recognizing spinal injuries

Spinal injuries, even serious ones, often do not show obvious signs and symptoms. Rely on the history of the scene, especially the mechanism of injury, to decide if there is a chance of a spinal injury. If the history of the scene suggests a spinal injury, give first aid for a spinal injury even if the

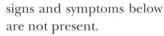

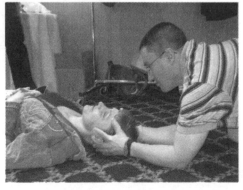

signs and symptoms below are not present.

6

Signs and symptoms of spinal injuries

◆ swelling and/or bruising at the site of the injury

◆ numbness, tingling or a loss of feeling in the arms and legs on one or both sides of the body

◆ not able to move arms and/or legs on one or both sides of the body

◆ pain at the injury site

◆ signs of shock (see page 67).

 ## Stabilization of a head or spinal injury

6

The aim of first aid for spinal injuries is to prevent further injury, especially to the spinal cord. Further injury is caused by moving the injured area. The first aid is to prevent spinal movement. When moving the casualty is necessary, support her in a way that minimizes movement of the head and spine.

1 Begin ESM—start the scene survey. As soon as you suspect a head or spinal injury, tell the casualty not to move.

2 Steady and support the casualty's head and neck as soon as you can—show a bystander how to do this. Show a second bystander how to steady and support the feet. The head and feet should be continuously supported until either the casualty is fully immobilized or medical help takes over.

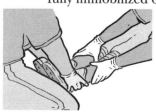 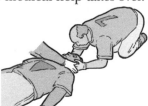

Keep elbows on the ground to keep your arms steady.

Firmly hold the head with fingers along the line of the jaw.

3   Assess responsiveness and then do a primary survey. If the casualty is unresponsive, check for breathing before opening the airway. If there is no breathing begin CPR with 30 compressions. After 30 initial compressions, open the airway using the head-tilt chin lift and give 2 ventilations. Continue CPR in cycles of 30 compressions followed by 2 ventilations.

Check circulation—look for signs of severe bleeding and shock.

4   Do a secondary survey to the extent needed, but do not move the casualty or poke and probe any possible spinal injury. If you suspect a pelvic injury, don't "test for it" by squeezing the hips together.

5   Decide whether you will need to transport the casualty. If medical help will arrive at the scene, it is probably best to steady and support the casualty in the position found and give ongoing casualty care. Continue to steady and support the head and feet until additional help arrives.

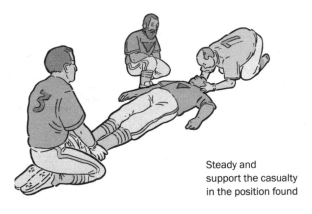

Steady and
support the casualty
in the position found

Pelvic injury

When you suspect a fractured pelvis, also suspect a spinal injury. If there was enough force to fracture the pelvis, the spine may also have been injured.

Signs and symptoms of pelvic injury

◆ signs of shock (casualty could be bleeding internally)

◆ casualty cannot stand or walk

◆ urge to urinate

◆ casualty cannot urinate or there is blood in the urine

◆ sharp pain in the groin and small of the back

◆ increased pain when moving

6

More on spine boards

A long spine board is usually the size shown below.

The long spine board is usually made of sturdy plastic. Holes along the sides and ends of the board serve as hand-holds. Straps and head hold may be pre-attached. Runners, tapered at each end and attached to the bottom of the board, make it easier to slide the board along rough surfaces. The runners also lift the board off the ground, making it easier to grasp the hand-holds.

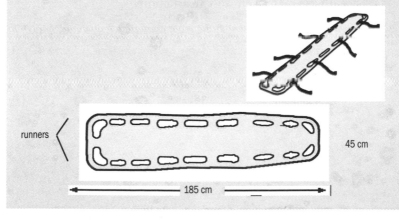

runners

45 cm

185 cm

Immobilizing a fractured pelvis

Give first aid as you would for a spinal injury (see page 249) but include the following:

◆ the pelvic area may not be stable—if you suspect a pelvic injury, do not squeeze the hips together when examining the casualty

◆ if medical help is coming to the scene, steady and support the casualty in the position found. Stabilize the pelvic area with heavy padding such as blankets

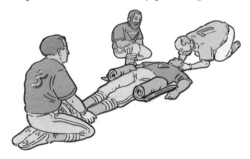

If the casualty will be transported, a scoop stretcher is needed to do this safely. Specific training is required. Procedures should be developed and practiced consistent with the manufacturer's instructions.

Possible complications the may result from a pelvic injury include injury to the lower spine and/or injury to the bladder that may lead to infection.

6

Rib or breastbone injury

Signs and symptoms

◆ pain at injury site when casualty moves, coughs or breathes deeply

◆ shallow breathing

◆ casualty guards injury

◆ deformity and discolouration

◆ may be a wound

◆ may cough up frothy blood (if lung punctured)

◆ may show signs of shock

Complications

◆ pneumothorax or tension pneumothorax

◆ punctured lung

◆ severe breathing difficulties

 First aid for injured ribs or breastbone

First aid for injured ribs or breastbone aims to reduce the chance of further injury, to minimize pain and to make breathing easier. Consider the mechanism of injury. If the force was sufficient to injure or fracture the breastbone, suspect a spinal injury and do not move the casualty.

1 Start ESM—do a scene survey. Do a primary survey. Give first aid for life-threatening injuries.

2 Expose the injured area and look for a wound. If there is a wound, check for a penetrating chest wound (see page 188). Put an appropriate dressing on the wound and get medical help quickly.

3   If injuries permit, place the casualty in a semi-sitting position, leaning slightly toward the injured side—this should help breathing. Hand support over the injured area may make breathing easier.

4   Support the arm on the injured side in a St. John tubular sling to transfer its weight to the uninjured side.

5   Give ongoing casualty care—monitor breathing often. Get medical help.

A fracture of one or two ribs is very painful and causes shallow breathing, but the casualty does not usually have severe breathing difficulties, or show signs of shock.

If severe breathing problems arise, refer to page 89.

Flail chest

A flail chest results when several ribs in the same area are broken in more than one place. The injured part of the chest wall is called a "flail" or "loose" segment. The flail segment is no longer a rigid part of the chest wall, so it doesn't move normally during breathing. As the casualty inhales, the chest should expand, but the flail segment is pulled into the chest instead. As the casualty exhales, the chest should move inward, but the flail segment puffs outward. This abnormal chest movement is called **paradoxical chest movement**. This injury makes breathing very difficult because of the pain and the tissue damage.

Signs and symptoms of a flail chest

◆ paradoxical chest movement—this is the sign that will tell you whether there is a flail chest

◆ breathing is very painful, and the casualty may be positioned to support the injured area

◆ bruising at the injury site

 First aid for a flail chest

The aim of first aid for a flail chest is to give first aid for the ABCs, immobilize the casualty and get medical help.

1   Begin ESM—do a scene survey. As soon as you suspect major injuries, tell the casualty not to move.

2   Steady and support the head and neck.

3   Start the primary survey—check airway and breathing.

4   If the casualty complains of difficulty breathing and pain in the chest, expose and examine the injury.

5   Support the injured area with your hand—this may make breathing easier.

6   Give first aid for ineffective breathing if needed (see page 98).

7   Check circulation and give first aid if needed.

8   Give ongoing casualty care until medical help takes over.

6

Pneumothorax–
a serious complication of a chest injury

The pleural space is the space between the lungs and the chest wall that is usually not a space at all—it is filled with the lungs. The lungs are sucked into this space because there is no air in it. But if air gets into the space, the lung on that side won't be sucked into it, and it will collapse. A pneumothorax (pronounced "new-mow-thor-ax") occurs when air gets into the pleural space. It is life-threatening because the lungs can collapse and cause the person severe breathing difficulties.

Open pneumothorax

An open pneumothorax occurs when there is a penetrating wound to the chest and air is going through the wound into the pleural space. It is called "open" because the pneumothorax is "open" to the outside through the wound. A penetrating chest wound is an open pneumothorax.

Closed pneumothorax

There doesn't have to be an external chest wound for a pneumothorax. Air can enter the pleural space from inside the body through a damaged lung or airway. This can happen by itself without any obvious cause (called a "spontaneous" pneumothorax), or from an injury, like a broken rib piercing the lung.

Tension pneumothorax

If air keeps going into the pleural space and can't get out, it builds up—this is a tension pneumothorax. As the air builds up, it collapses the lung and puts pressure on the heart which then can't pump blood as well as it should. If the air keeps building up, the casualty's condition will worsen. A tension pneumothorax is a serious medical emergency.

Sealing a penetrating chest wound with an airtight dressing can cause a tension pneumothorax. If there is also a wound inside the chest, air can get into the chest cavity through the lung or airway, but it can't get out because you've sealed the wound, so it builds up. This is where the flutter-valve of the sucking chest wound dressing is important. It allows the air building up inside the chest to escape as the casualty exhales, but it doesn't let air into the chest as the casualty inhales (see page 188).

If air is getting into the chest cavity through a damaged lung, and there is no chest wound, the first aider cannot stop any build-up of air in the pleural space. Get medical help as quickly as possible and make the casualty as comfortable as you can.

Pneumothorax

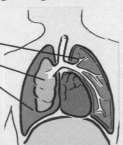

normal lung

collapsed lung

air has entered the space between the lungs and chest wall and caused the lung to collapse—this is a pneumothorax

Tension pneumothorax

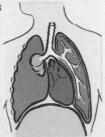

air is building up in the chest cavity on the injured side

the air puts pressure on the heart and other lung—this is a tension pneumothorax

Collarbone/shoulder blade fracture

Signs and symptoms

◆ pain at injury site

◆ swelling and deformity

◆ loss of function of the arm on the side of the injury

◆ casualty holds and protects the arm if he can, and may tilt the head to the injured side

Possible complications

◆ circulation to the arm below the injury may be impaired or cut off

6

 Immobilizing a collarbone or shoulder blade

The collarbone (clavicle) and shoulder blade (scapula) form and support the shoulder. These bones can be fractured by either direct force, like a blow to the shoulder, or by indirect force like falling on an outstretched hand. Immobilize the injury as shown below.

1 Check circulation below the injury. If circulation is impaired, get medical help quickly.

2 Immobilize the arm in the position of most comfort. A St. John tubular sling may work well (see page 166).

St. John
tubular sling
transfers the
weight of the
arm to the
uninjured
side

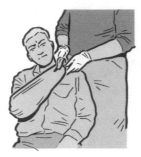
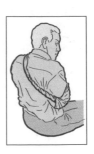

3   Secure the arm to the chest with a broad bandage to
prevent movement of the arm. Pad under the elbow,
if necessary, to keep the arm in the most comfortable
position. Tie the bandage on the uninjured side—
don't tie it so tightly that the arm is pulled out of
position. Pad under the knots for comfort.

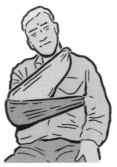

4   Check circulation below the injury. If circulation is
impaired, and it was not before, loosen the sling and
bandage.

Immobilizing a dislocated joint

Padding, bandages, slings and splints may be used to immobilize a dislocation. Usually the dislocated joint won't move very easily in any direction, and any movement causes pain. Immobilize the limb in the position of most comfort—usually the position found.

The following illustrations show suggestions for immobilizing a dislocated shoulder, or the casualty may want to hold the injured arm herself. If the casualty's arm will bend into position for a St. John tubular sling, this may be the most comfortable position.

If the arm will bend:

◆ use a St. John tubular sling to transfer the weight of the arm to the other side (see page 166)

◆ use broad bandages to prevent movement

◆ pad under the elbow for support

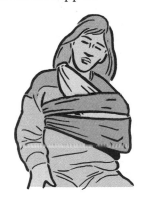

If the arm will not bend

◆ support the weight of the arm with a bandage around the neck

◆ bandage the arm to the body to prevent movement

◆ pad under the elbow, if necessary, to keep the arm in the most comfortable position

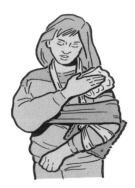

The success of the method you use depends on whether it stops the injured limb from moving—which causes pain and could cause further injury. Often, the "trick" is to use just the right amount of padding between the arm and body so the bandages hold the arm in the most comfortable position. Tie the bandages securely but not so tightly they put pressure on the injured limb.

Once the injury is immobilized, apply cold to help reduce pain and swelling (see page 238) providing the casualty can tolerate the added weight.

Monitor circulation below the injury often—check the skin colour and temperatureuse the nailbed test and check for a pulse. Compare the injured side with the uninjured side. If circulation becomes impaired after immobilizing the injury, loosen the bandages. If circulation remains impaired, get medical help quickly.

6

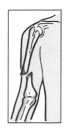

Immobilizing the upper arm

The following shows how to immobilize an open fracture of the upper arm (humerus). Immobilize a closed fracture of the upper arm as shown in step 3.

1 Expose the injury site. Cover the wound with a sterile dressing and check circulation. See page 275 for more on dressing an open fracture wound.

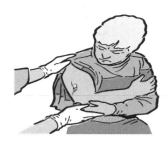
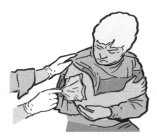

2 Pad and bandage the dressings. Pad lengthwise on both sides of the fracture site. Padding should be bulky enough to protect any protruding bone ends. Hold padding in place with tape if needed.

Bandage dressings tightly enough to hold padding and dressings in place. The bandage shouldn't put any pressure on bone ends.

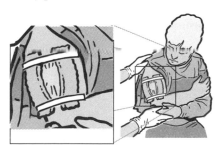
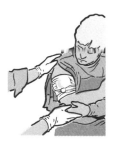

3   Immobilize the arm with a sling (see page 165) and broad bandages. An arm sling provides full support for the arm—broad bandages above and below fracture site prevent arm movement. Pad under the elbow as needed to hold the arm in the position of comfort.

Injured elbow

Signs and symptoms

◆ pain at injury site

◆ swelling and deformity

◆ loss of function of the arm on the side of the injury

◆ casualty holds and protects the injury

Complications

◆ circulation and/or nerve function to the arm below the injury could be impaired or cut off

Immobilizing an injured elbow

The elbow can be severely sprained, fractured or dislocated. Immobilize the injury in the position found, if possible, or in the position of greatest comfort.

1   Expose the injury and look for any open wounds. Check circulation below the injury and compare it with the other side. If circulation is impaired, get medical help quickly.

2 If the elbow is bent so the arm is in front of the chest, immobilize the arm in an arm sling (see page 161).

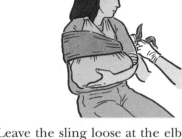

Leave the sling loose at the elbow. Pad under the elbow, if necessary, to keep the arm in the most comfortable position and use a broad bandage to limit movement.

3 If the elbow will not bend, support the arm at the wrist and use broad bandages and padding to immobilize the arm.

Place broad bandages above and below the injury.

Check circulation below the injury and compare it with the other side—if it is impaired, and it wasn't before, adjust the sling and/or bandages.

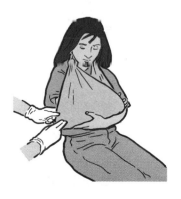
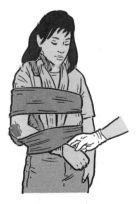

Splinting materials

Definition

A splint is any material used to prevent fractured bones from moving unnecessarily. Fractured arms, hands, fingers, legs, feet and toes can all be splinted.

A good splint is. . .

◆ rigid enough to support the injured limb

◆ well padded for support and comfort

◆ long enough, which means:

◆   – for a fracture between 2 joints, it extends beyond the joints above and below the fracture

◆   – for an injured joint, it's long enough for the limb to be secured so the joint can't move

There are many commercial splints available. You may have access to one of these if the incident happened at a workplace, sporting event, etc. Training is required before using these splints. Always follow the manufacturer's directions.

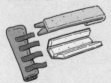
Commercial splints

A splint can be improvised from any material, as long as it works to immobilize the injury.

The casualty's own body can be used as a splint. One leg can be splinted to the other. Fingers and toes can be splinted to the next finger or toe. This is called an "anatomical" splint.

Other materials needed for splinting

To put the splint on you will need materials for padding and bandages.

Padding does two things:

◆ it fills in the natural hollows between the body and the splint, ensuring the injured limb is properly supported

◆ it makes the splint more comfortable

Always pad between a splint and the injured limb, and between two body parts to be bandaged together.

Bandages are used to secure the splint to the body. If you have triangular bandages, fold and use them as broad bandages (see page 159). When using bandages:

◆ make sure they are wide enough to provide firm support without discomfort

◆ pass them under the natural hollows of the body—go under the knee, the small of the back, the hollow behind the ankles

◆ tie them tightly enough to prevent movement, but not so tight they cut off circulation. Check circulation every 15 minutes below any bandages you've tied

Improvised splints

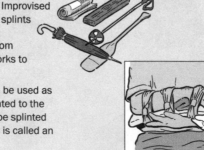

General information on splinting

Splinting helps prevent:

◆ movement of the broken bones

◆ further damage to soft tissues like nerves, the spinal cord and blood vessels

◆ a closed fracture from becoming an open fracture

◆ impaired circulation below the injury

◆ excessive bleeding into the tissues at the fracture site

Splinting also:

◆ helps to reduce pain

◆ makes transporting the casualty easier

When splinting:

◆ expose the injury before splinting so you can fully assess it

◆ check circulation below the injury both before and after splinting

◆ if not sure whether to splint an injury, splint it

◆ dress and bandage any wounds before splinting

◆ realign a severely deformed limb before splinting if circulation is impaired

◆ before putting a splint on, measure it against the uninjured limb

◆ don't cover wounds with splints, if possible

◆ only use commercial splints if you are trained in their use

◆ after splinting, check all the bandages and the circulation below the last bandage

6

When is medical help needed?

It is always safest to get medical help for any injury. Injuries that appear minor can be more serious than they seem, and minor injuries can benefit from medical treatment.

First aiders may be in the awkward position of trying to convince a casualty to get medical help. The following points indicate when all activity should be stopped and medical help consulted.

Stop activity and get medical help when:

◆ there is any loss in the range of motion, meaning the injured area doesn't move the way it usually does

◆ the casualty complains of pain during normal activity. This means if the casualty limps, favours the injured side, or shows any sign of injury, medical help should be consulted

◆ there is a loss of circulation below the injury.

Immobilizing the forearm and wrist

Immobilize the forearm and wrist as shown below when you suspect the forearm or wrist is fractured, or the wrist is badly sprained.

1   Examine the injury and decide the best position for splinting—this is usually in the position found. Have the casualty or a bystander steady and support the injured arm as you gather and prepare the supplies you will need.

2   Measure the splint against the uninjured arm to make sure it is the right size. Pad the splint for comfort and to support the fracture. Position the arm on the splint with as little movement as possible.

fractured forearm

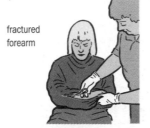

fractured wrist

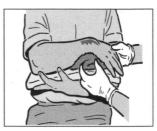

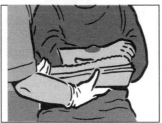

This splint extends from beyond the elbow to the fingers, and is padded along the full length for firm support of the fractured arm

This splint supports the elbow, forearm and hand, and is padded to keep the fractured wrist in the position found

3 Once the splint is in position, have the casualty or bystander support it while you secure the splint.

With a roller bandage, start above the injury. Wrap the splint and the arm snugly, but not too tightly. Wrap enough of the arm above and below the injury to immobilize the fracture. Leave the fingertips visible so you can check circulation below the injury and bandages.

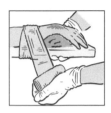
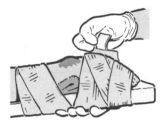
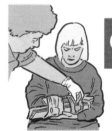

Secure the splint with broad bandages above and below the injury. Tuck in any loose ends.

4 Use an arm sling to support the lower arm and hand, and prevent movement of the elbow. Fingertips are exposed so you can check circulation below the injury and bandages. Tie the sling so the arm is slightly elevated.

5 Check circulation below the last bandage. If circulation is impaired, and it wasn't before, loosen the sling and bandage. If circulation remains impaired, get medical help urgently.

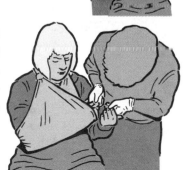

Immobilizing an injured hand

Immobilize an injured hand as shown below when you suspect bones in the hand are fractured.

1   Examine the injured hand and decide the best position for splinting—this is usually in the position of function (see opposite page). Have the casualty or a bystander steady and support the injury as you gather and prepare the supplies you will need. If there are open wounds, place non-stick sterile dressings between the fingers to prevent the fingers sticking together.

2   Measure the splint against the uninjured hand and arm to make sure it is the right size. Position the arm on the splint with as little movement as possible. The illustrations below and on the next page show two types of splints, a pillow and a board.

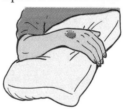

Using a pillow

A pillow works well because it lets the hand rest in the position of function and it is padded but also firm. It fully supports the wrist and lower arm.

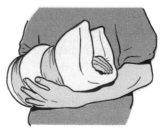

◆ secure the pillow with 2 broad bandages, making sure there is no pressure on the hand.

◆ leave fingertips visible to check for circulation

Using a board

A board works well because it is rigid, but, you must use padding to keep the hand in the position of function.

♦ secure the splint with a roller bandage. Leave fingertips visible to check for circulation.

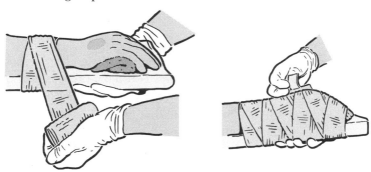

6

3   Immobilize the arm in an arm sling tied to keep the lower arm and hand slightly elevated (see page 165). Check circulation in the fingers.

Position of function

The position of function is the position the uninjured hand naturally takes—palm down and fingers slightly curled. This position is safer and more comfortable than trying to flatten the hand against a flat surface.

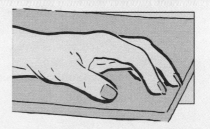

Immobilizing an injured finger or thumb

Immobilize a fractured or dislocated finger or thumb in the position found.

1   Expose the injury. Check the circulation below the injury.

2   Immobilize the finger or thumb in the position of most comfort, which is usually the position of function. Use a splint, as shown below, or if a splint is not available, secure the injured finger or thumb to the uninjured finger beside it.

Fractured finger   Fractured thumb

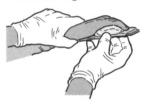
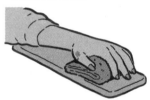

Use padding to provide extra support.

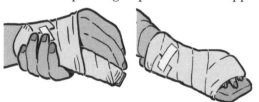

3   Put on a St John tubular sling (see page 166) to keep the injury elevated. Be careful not to put pressure on the injury. Check circulation below the injury.

4   Give ongoing casualty care and get medical help.

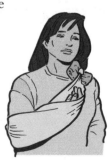

Fractured upper leg (femur)

Signs and symptoms

◆ pain, perhaps severe

◆ the foot and leg roll outward

◆ deformity and shortening of the leg

Possible complications

◆ there can be internal bleeding, causing severe shock

Immobilizing an injured upper leg (femur)

neck of the femur

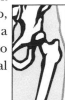

A common fracture of the upper leg is a break at the neck of the femur. This is often referred to as a broken hip, and most commonly happens to elderly people during a fall. In a younger, healthy person, great force is needed to fracture the upper leg—always assess for a head or spinal injury.

1 If you suspect a fractured upper leg, have a bystander steady and support the injured limb.

Choose one of the splinting techniques on the next page. In either case:

2 Gather the splinting materials. Measure the splint(s) against the uninjured leg. Put bandages into position. Pad the splints and position them as shown.

3 Tie the bandages from chest to ankle—from the stable end to the unstable end.

4 Give ongoing casualty care. Get medical help.

6

Using a long splint only   **Using a long and a short splint**

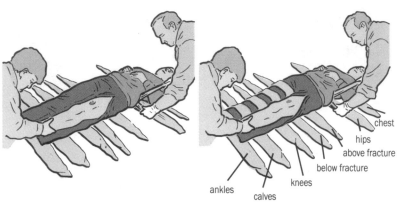

chest
hips
above fracture
below fracture
knees
calves
ankles

Push bandages under the natural hollows of the body and position as shown above.

Splint placed just below the armpit

Position the inside splint just below groin

Outside splint placed just below armpit

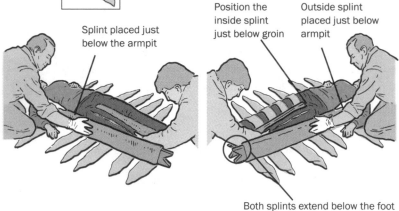

Both splints extend below the foot

All bandages are tied off on the splint

Steady and support until this figure-8 bandage is tied

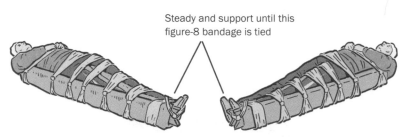

Immobilizing an injured knee

Have a bystander steady and support the injured leg. Expose and assess the injury. If the leg is straight, splint a shown below. If the leg is bent, try to straighten it. Depending on the injury, the casualty may be able to straighten the leg with your help. With a more severe injury, gently move the leg into a straightened position.

Don't try to straighten the leg if the pain increases or the leg does not move easily. If the leg won't straighten easily or without increased pain, splint in the position found.

If the leg is straight

If the leg is bent

6

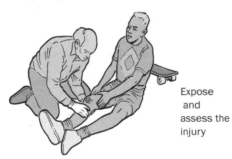

Expose and assess the injury

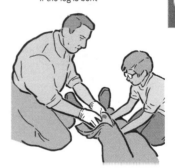

Carefully lift the injured leg and position a padded splint

Position five broad bandages under the leg—two above the knee and three below

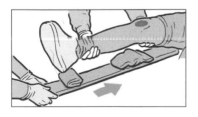

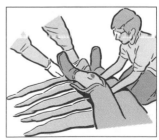

Adjust the pads to fit the natural hollows of the leg

Position padded splints on the inside and outside of the leg

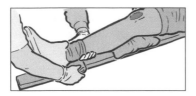

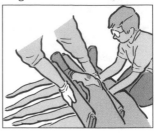

Position 2 broad bandages and secure the splint to the leg -use a figure-8 at the ankle

Secure the splint with the bandages, keeping the leg in the bent position

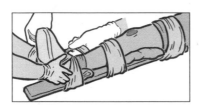

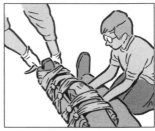

6

Immobilizing an open fracture of the lower leg (tibia and/or fibula)

A fractured lower leg is a common sports injury. The example here shows an open fracture. Immobilize a closed fracture the same way but without the dressings and bandages over the wound.

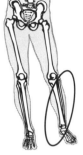

1 Expose the injury. Clothing is removed by cutting to minimize movement of the injured leg. Here the first aider discovers the injury is an open fracture.

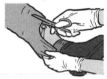
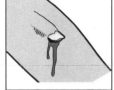

a fracture is "open" when the skin is broken—the bone may stick out

6

2 Show a bystander how to steady and support the leg. Check the circulation below the injury. Give first aid for the open fracture wound. Leave the shoe on unless there is a wound to be examined.

Cover the wound with a sterile dressing.

Dressing an open fracture

When there is an open fracture, give first aid for the wound first and then immobilize the fracture. For the wound, apply a sterile dressing to prevent further contamination. To stop bleeding from the wound, apply pressure around the fracture, but not on it. Apply a dressing with padding on both sides of the fracture site. Secure this with a broad bandage tied tightly enough to put pressure on the padding. Always check circulation before and after dressing a wound of this type.

6

The dressing should extend well beyond the edges of the wound. Put bulky padding lengthwise on both sides of the fracture, over the dressing, to protect the bone end.

It may help to tape the padding in place.

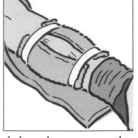

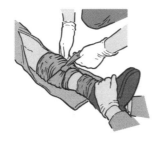

Tie a broad bandage over the padding and dressing tightly enough to put pressure on the padding, but not tight enough to cut off circulation—check circulation below the injury once the bandage is tied. Make sure there is no pressure on the bone ends.

3 Immobilize the lower leg. Position the bandages and splints. Use two padded splints long enough to extend from the groin to below the foot. The bystander doesn't let go of the leg until the first aider tells him to, which is after the last bandage is tied. Tie all knots on the splint for comfort.

Position broad bandages to be tied at the:

thigh
knee
above the fracture
below the fracture
ankle

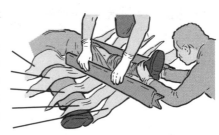

4   Tie the bandages starting at the thigh (the stable end) and working down. The bandage at the ankles is tied as a figure-8.

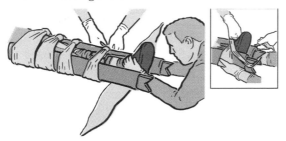

5   Check the circulation below the injury, elevate the injured leg and give ongoing casualty care. Get medical help.

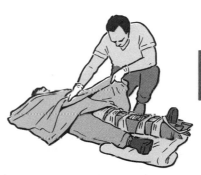

6

If you don't have splints ...

Use the uninjured leg as an **anatomical** splint by tying the legs together.

Position padding between the legs (rolled up blanket).

Position and tie broad bandages at the thighs, knees, above the injury, below the injury and at the ankles. Tie a figure-8 at the ankles.

Tie knots on padding for comfort.

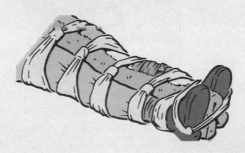

Immobilizing an injured ankle

The ankle should be immobilized whenever you suspect a sprain or a fracture. If you suspect a serious injury, including an open fracture, immobilize the lower leg as shown on page 275. If the injury doesn't seem serious, or if the journey to medical help will be smooth, use a blanket splint or pillow splint to immobilize the ankle, as shown below.

1   Check circulation below the injury. If circulation is impaired (see page 175).

2   Loosen footwear and immobilize the ankle. Position a pillow or rolled-up blanket and two broad bandages. Make sure the splint extends beyond the ankle.

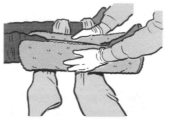

Secure the pillow with two broad bandages—use a figure-8 at the ankle.

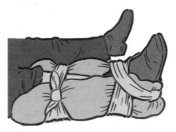

3   Check circulation below the injury. Elevate the injured limb and apply cold (see RICE, page 238). Give ongoing casualty care and get medical help.

Immobilizing an injured foot or toe

1 Check circulation below the injury. If circulation is impaired, get medical help quickly.

2 Immobilize the ankle using a double figure-8.

Untie shoe laces and tie the first figure-8 beginning at the sole of the foot and tying toward the leg.

Tie the second figure-8 by wrapping the ends around the leg, crossing in front of the ankle and tying off on the sole of the foot.

Tie off at the sole.

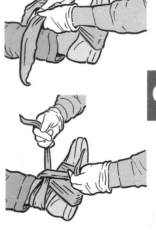

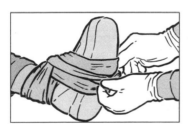

Every few minutes ask the casualty if the bandage feels tight—this may happen as the injured area swells.

Immobilizing a toe

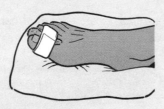

Immobilize a fractured toe by taping it to the uninjured toe beside it.

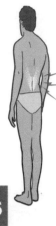

Strains

When a muscle or tendon is over-stretched or forcefully shortened, it can result in a stretch or tear injury, called a strain.   There are different degrees of strains, from mildly uncomfortable to disabling, but it is difficult for a first aider to determine the exact degree of a strain. Muscles strains of the lower back are common.

Signs and symptoms

The signs and symptoms of a strain often show up many hours after the injury.

◆ sudden sharp pain in the strained muscle

◆ swelling of the muscles causing severe cramps (e.g. charley horse)

◆ bruising and muscle stiffness

◆ casualty may not be able to use the affected body part (loss of function)

 ### First aid for strains

1   Begin ESM—do a scene survey. Have the casualty stop the activity that caused the injury.

2   Place the casualty in a position of comfort and assess the injury. If there is loss of function, immobilize the injury as for a fracture. Use RICE (see page 238).

3   Give ongoing casualty care. Get medical help. Position the casualty on his back with knees raised to   take pressure off lower back muscles.

Preventing bone, joint and muscle injuries

Preventing fractures

Most fractures can be prevented by adopting good safety habits.

Motor vehicle collisions are the cause of many bone injuries. Defensive driving reduces the number of collisions, and the use of seat belts decreases the incidence and severity of injuries.

Adopt a what if attitude to every hazardous condition in the workplace and at home. Potential falls exist on every working and walking surface. Prevent the fall—avoid the injury. Ask yourself:

◆ what if work areas are cluttered and untidy? What if tools, hoses, extension cords are left lying about?

◆ what if floors are wet, greasy and slippery? What if floor coverings—carpets, rugs at the tops and bottoms of stairs, tiles and floorboards are loose?

◆ what if stairs are poorly lit, cluttered with shoes, toys or newspapers, have no handrails, are covered with ice and snow? What if chairs are used to reach high places, stepladders are in poor repair, ladders are not secured?

◆ what if life-lines and safety belts are not used when working in high places? What if children are left unattended on balconies?

The appropriate safety action in each of the above situations will take only a moment, but could save someone many days, weeks or months of pain and suffering from a preventable fall.

Preventing strains, sprains and dislocations

Strains, sprains and dislocations are caused by sudden excessive pulling or twisting of a muscle or joint. Strains or sprains are often the result of poor body mechanics or of inadequate conditioning of the body for a particular sport or physical activity. Dislocations are usually caused by violent movements.

◆ use proper body mechanics when lifting (see page 78)

◆ if you are not sure if you can manage lifting a load or moving a heavy object, don't try, get help

◆ warm up before exercising and don't push your limits while exercising

6

Repetitive strain injury (RSI)

Muscles and tendons can be injured when they do the same movements over and over again, especially when the movement causes stress on the tissues. These injuries develop over a period of time—days, weeks or months—but can be very disabling.

RSI injuries are also called overuse injuries; examples include tennis elbow, bursitis and carpal tunnel syndrome.

First aid for RSI

◆ stop the activity causing the injury

◆ refer the casualty to medical help

Immobilization of a head or spinal injury

In most instances you will stabilize the casualty and wait for medical help to arrive. It is possible that you will have to transport the casualty in the case where medical help is not available or will be delayed for hours. These steps involve advanced skills and specific training is recommended. The following steps pick up from step 5 on page 250.

1   If medical help will be delayed, or is not available, immobilize the casualty onto a spine board. Gather the materials and people you will need to immobilize the casualty when help arrives—see bottom of this page.

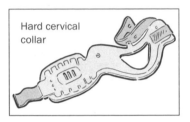

Hard cervical collar

2   If you have a hard cervical collar, and are trained to apply it, use it to immobilize the head and neck (see opposite page).

Materials for spinal immobilization

◆ hard cervical collar and oropharyngeal airway (OPA)
◆ a full-length spine board or other rigid flat surface like a door or piece of plywood
◆ at least 12 triangular bandages or straps, etc.
◆ at least 1 blanket plus two small pillows or another blanket
◆ 4 people plus yourself

Using hard cervical collars

The best way to immobilize the head and neck is to use a hard cervical collar. When a hard cervical collar is put on a casualty who is not fully conscious, or is at risk of losing consciousness, additional equipment is needed to keep the airway open. A first aider may use this equipment **if she is properly trained** and has the right equipment, in the correct sizes, available.

Hard cervical collars

The hard cervical collars used by emergency personnel, including first aiders, are especially designed for use at emergency scenes. Although they are quite simple, you need special training before using them. With training, you will learn:

◆ how to choose the right size collar

◆ how to properly move the head to align it with the neck

◆ how to put the collar on

◆ complications that may arise when using a hard cervical collar

There are different manufacturers of hard cervical collars and you should have training for the specific brand of collar you will be using.

Hard cervical collars and the airway

Before using a hard cervical collar, consider the casualty's airway. Remember that if the casualty is not fully conscious, the tongue may fall back and block the airway—and with a hard cervical collar, you won't be able to use the jaw-thrust, or even tilt the head back, to open the airway. To keep the airway open when using a

hard cervical collar you need to use an oropharyngeal airway (OPA).

An OPA is a device medical professionals use to keep an unconscious person's airway open. When properly sized and inserted, an OPA prevents the tongue from blocking

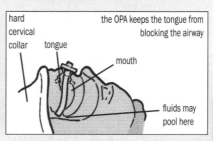

hard cervical collar   tongue   the OPA keeps the tongue from blocking the airway   mouth   fluids may pool here

the airway. However, even with an OPA, saliva and other fluids may pool in the back of the throat and block the airway. The only way to remove this fluid, while keeping the casualty face up, is with suction equipment designed specifically for use with an OPA. Only use an OPA when you have suctioning equipment available.

When to use a hard cervical collar and OPA

First, only use this equipment if you are trained. The points below note when to use what equipment:

◆ if the casualty is fully conscious and there is no head injury or other risk of losing consciousness, use a hard cervical collar even if you don't have an OPA

◆ if the casualty is not fully conscious, or has an injury that could cause loss of consciousness, only use a hard cervical collar if you have an OPA and appropriate suctioning equipment

6

3 Place the casualty on the spine board using the logroll, a method of rolling a casualty onto his side so the whole body moves as a unit. This reduces the chance of further tissue damage. Get the casualty ready by tying his wrists and legs together. This makes it much easier to roll him as a unit.

As you are preparing the casualty for transportation, keep talking to him, explaining what you are doing and why.

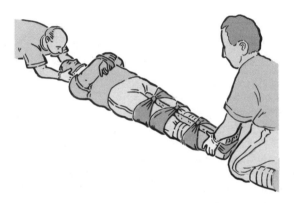

4 Position the prepared spine board beside the casualty. Position the assisting rescuers and yourself (first aider) as follows.

◆ you, the first aider, will pay particular attention to the neck and upper back for the entire procedure

◆ rescuers should already be positioned at the body and the feet

◆ position a rescuer beside you at the casualty's shoulder hips and upper legs

◆ if you have another rescuer, she can be positioned beside the spine board, ready to move it into position.

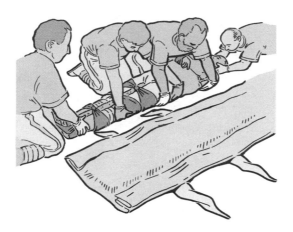

5 Give detailed instructions on how the logroll will proceed:

◆ tell the rescuers at the body and the feet that on the command, "roll," they will lift and turn the head and feet as the rest of the body rolls, so that the whole body turns as a unit

◆ tell the rescuer beside you that on the command, "roll," he will roll the casualty toward himself, using a firm grip to control the casualty

◆ tell the rescuer at the spine board that on the command, "spine board," she will position the spine board alongside the casualty.

◆ tell the group that when the spine board is in position, you will give the command, "roll," and slowly but firmly, you will all roll the casualty back onto the spine board

Emphasize that the casualty must always be turned as a unit. Ask the rescuers if there are any questions.

6   Tell the rescuers to get ready, making sure each has a good, firm grip on the casualty. Logroll the casualty and position the spine board.

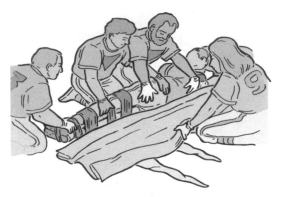

6

7   When the spine board is properly positioned, direct the bearers to roll the casualty back onto the board. Position the casualty in the centre of the spine board by pulling on the blanket.

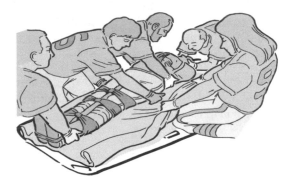

8 When the casualty is positioned on the spine board, pad around the head and wrap the blanket around him. Secure him to the spine board with narrow bandages and/or ties.

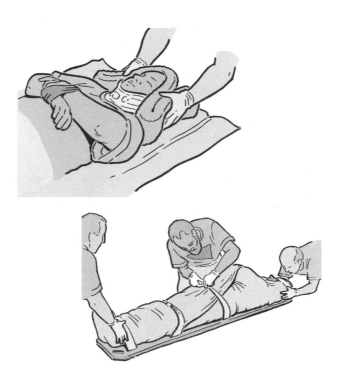

9 Give ongoing casualty care—monitor breathing often. Get medical help quickly and as smoothly as possible. Carry the spine board as explained on page 89.

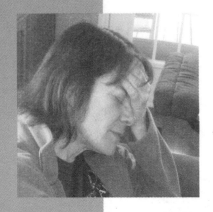

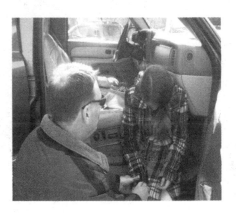

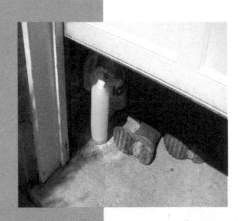

CHAPTER 7

ADDITIONAL FIRST AID EMERGENCIES

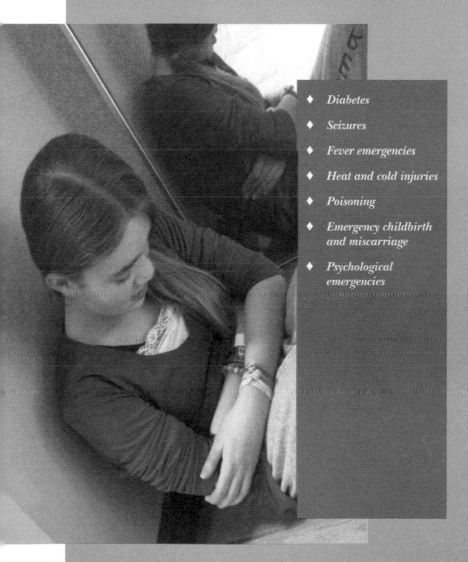

- ◆ *Diabetes*
- ◆ *Seizures*
- ◆ *Fever emergencies*
- ◆ *Heat and cold injuries*
- ◆ *Poisoning*
- ◆ *Emergency childbirth and miscarriage*
- ◆ *Psychological emergencies*

Diabetes

In a healthy person, the body produces the insulin needed to allow cells to take up sugar and convert the sugar into energy. Diabetes is a condition in which there is either not enough insulin in the blood or there is enough insulin but the cells cannot use the insulin properly. As a result, sugar builds up in the blood, and the cells don't get the energy they need.

hypoglycemia—not enough sugar, too much insulin

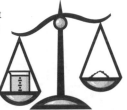

hyperglycemia—too much sugar, not enough insulin

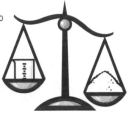

A person with diabetes may take medication by mouth or injection, and carefully controls what she eats (the source of energy) and her level of exercise (the use of energy). A diabetic emergency occurs when there is too much or too little insulin in the blood.

Causes, signs and symptoms of diabetic emergencies

	hypoglycemia (needs sugar)	hyeprglycemia (needs insulin)
time to develop	develops very quickly	develops over hours or days
possible cause	- took too much insulin - not eaten enough, or vomited - more exercise than usual	- did not take enough insulin - eating too much food - less exercise than usual - casualty has an ongoing illness and her body needs more insulin
pulse/breathing	strong and rapid/shallow	weak and rapid/deep and sighing
skin condition	sweaty, pale and cold	flushed, dry and warm
level of consc.	faintness to unconscious	drowsy, becoming unconscious
other signs and symptoms	- headache - confused, irritable and aggressive - trembling, staggering - difficulty speaking	- thirsty, then nausea and vomiting - frequent urination - breath has a nail polish smell

First aid for diabetic emergencies

It is important for first aiders to recognize the casualty's condition as an emergency. The aim of first aid in a diabetic emergency is to keep the casualty's condition from getting worse while you get medical help.

1 Begin ESM—do a scene survey. If the casualty is unresponsive, get medical help immediately.

2 Do a primary survey and give first aid for the ABCs.

3 After providing first aid for life-threatening conditions:

if the casualty is unconscious, place her into the recovery position and monitor the ABCs until medical help takes over. The casualty may be wearing a medical alert device that will give you more information about her condition.

if the casualty is conscious, ask what is wrong. She may be able to tell you, or she may be confused.

❖ if the casualty can tell you what she needs, or if you can tell by the signs and symptoms, help her take what is needed— usually this is sugar.

❖ if the casualty is confused about what is needed, give her something sweet to eat or drink—sugar may help, and if it does not, it will not make the casualty any worse

Sweeten a drink with 30 ml (2 tablespoons) of sugar or give something else sweet, like apple juice. Diet soft drinks will not help.

If the casualty is conscious and very weak, place her in the position of most comfort.

4   Give ongoing casualty care. Send for medical help if you have not done so already.

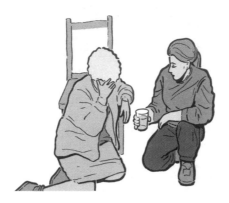

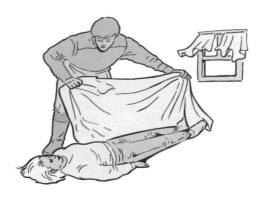

Don't confuse a diabetic emergency with drunkenness. Many of the behavioural signs are the same, but a person having a diabetic emergency needs immediate medical help. Check the signs and look for a medical alert device.

Seizures and convulsions

A seizure is caused by abnormal electrical activity in the brain. In a partial seizure, only part of the brain is affected. The person may experience a tingling or twitching in one area of the body. In a generalized seizure, the whole brain is affected—the person loses consciousness and may have convulsions. A convulsion is an abnormal muscle contraction, or series of muscle contractions, that the person cannot control.

Epilepsy is a disorder of the nervous system characterized by seizures. Many people with seizure disorders like epilepsy take medication to control the condition. Other causes of seizures include:

- head or brain injury
- brain infection
- a high fever in infants and children
- stroke
- drug overdose

7

With epilepsy, the person may feel that a seizure is about to occur because of a brief sensation she experiences, called an aura. The aura, which may be a hallucinated sound, smell, or a feeling of movement in the body, is felt just before the seizure.

A typical generalized seizure has two phases:

The "tonic" phase involves a sudden loss of consciousness causing the person to fall. The person's body becomes rigid for up to a minute during which the face and neck may turn bluish.

In the "clonic" phase, convulsions occur, breathing is noisy, frothy saliva may appear around the mouth and the teeth may grind.

A major seizure can come on very suddenly, but seldom lasts longer than three minutes.

When the seizure is over, the muscles gradually relax and the person regains consciousness. After the seizure, the person may not remember what happened. She may appear dazed and confused, and feel exhausted and sleepy.

Signs and symptoms of a generalized seizure

◆ a sudden cry, stiffening of the body and loss of consciousness causing the person to fall

◆ noisy breathing and frothy saliva at the mouth

◆ the body jerks

◆ breathing may stop or be irregular for a minute—the casualty may turn blue

◆ loss of bladder and bowel control

 ### First aid for a seizure or convulsion

First aid for a seizure aims to protect the casualty from injury during convulsions and to keep the airway open while the casualty is unconscious.

1 Begin ESM—do a scene survey. Make the area safe—clear away hard or sharp objects that could cause injury. Clear onlookers away to ensure the casualty's privacy.

During convulsions:

◆ don't restrict the casualty's movements. Gently guide them, if necessary, to protect from injury

◆ carefully loosen tight clothing, especially around the neck

◆ place something soft under the head

◆ do not try to put anything in the mouth, between the teeth or to hold the tongue

After convulsions:

◆ assess responsiveness and do a primary survey. Place the unconscious casualty into the recovery position—wipe away any fluids from the mouth and nose

2 Do a secondary survey to see if the casualty was injured during the seizure (although it is rare, injury is possible)—give first aid for any injuries.

3 Give ongoing casualty care, monitoring breathing, keeping the casualty warm and allowing her to rest (she may need up to an hour).

◆ don't give the casualty any liquids during or immediately after a seizure

Call for medical help if:

◆ the casualty is unconscious for more than five minutes, or has a second major seizure within a few minutes

◆ this is the person's first seizure or the cause of the seizure is unknown (ask the casualty when she regains consciousness)

Fever emergencies in infants and children

A rapid rise in temperature to 40°C (104°F) or higher can cause convulsions in infants and children. A fever emergency is when the temperature, taken in the armpit, is:

◆ 38°C (100.5°F) or higher for an infant

   40°C (104°F) or higher for a child

First aid for a fever emergency in an infant or child

1   Begin ESM—do a scene survey.

2   Advise the parent/caregiver to call the doctor immediately and follow her advice. If the doctor can't be reached, advise the parent/caregiver to give acetaminophen (e.g. Tempra® or Tylenol®) or children's ibuprofen (not ASA—see warning below) according to the directions on the label. This should bring down the child's temperature.

Do not give ASA (e.g. Aspirin®) to children or adolescents because it may cause Reye's syndrome, a life-threatening condition.

Do not use cold water when sponging the child—this may cause more serious problems. Only use lukewarm water.

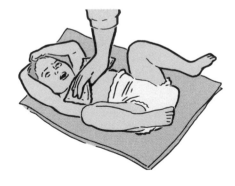

3   Encourage the fully conscious child to drink fluids.

4   If the temperature doesn't go down, sponge the child with lukewarm water for about 20 minutes. Don't immerse the child or infant in a tub—the temperature will go down more quickly if the wet skin is exposed to air currents.

5   Dry and dress the child in comfortable but not overly warm clothing. Monitor the child's temperature and repeat steps 3 to 5, as necessary, until medical help is reached.

6   If the child has a convulsion:

◆ don't restrain the child, but protect her from injury by removing hard objects and gently guiding movements

◆ loosen constrictive clothing

7   When the convulsions stop, perform a primary survey.

8   Give ongoing care, place the child into the best recovery position for her age (see page 61).

Cold Related Injuries

How the body loses heat

Core body temperature drops when the body loses more heat than it produces. There are five ways the body loses heat. The table on page 299 explains each of these. In an outdoor emergency, heat loss by conduction and convection (wet and wind) are often the main contributors to hypothermia. But when trying to prevent heat loss, you must look for all the ways the body is losing heat.

How the body adapts to heat loss

The body has a number of ways to minimize heat loss and keep the body core warm. One of the first things the body does when it is losing heat is start shivering. The muscle action of shivering generates heat. By shivering, the body is trying to warm itself. If the body keeps getting colder, the blood vessels in the arms, legs and at the skin surface get smaller. This keeps the blood in the core, where it is warmest. By doing this, the body core uses the surface tissues to insulate itself from the cold.

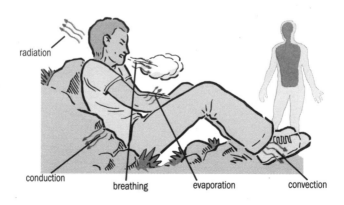

radiation

conduction   breathing   evaporation   convection

If heat loss continues, the body processes get slower. This includes thinking, muscular action and the senses. Shivering will become uncontrollable and then will slow down and eventually stop. The muscles get stiff and movements become jerky. Thinking is confused, speech difficult and the senses dulled. The heart and breathing rates slow down and the person eventually loses consciousness. At this point, the condition is very serious. The heartbeat becomes unsteady and faint, and finally the heart stops.

When the heart stops beating, the person is considered dead. However, when body tissues are cold, they aren't damaged as easily by a lack of oxygen. For this reason, there is often a chance of resuscitating a hypothermic person who doesn't show any signs of life. This means that as long as you aren't putting yourself or others at risk, you should continue your rescue efforts to get a hypothermic casualty to medical help.

7

How the body loses heat, examples and prevention

Heat loss	Explanation	Example	Sample prevention
1. Radiation	Heat radiates from the body into the air around it.	A lot of heat radiates from the skin.	Wear warm clothes.
2. Breathing	Cold air is inhaled, warmed by the body and exhaled, causing heat loss.	The steam you see when you exhale on a cold day is cold air that your body has just warmed, and lost heat in doing so.	Wear a parka with a "tunnel" hood or "ski-tube"—the air you breath will be warmer than the outside air.
3. Evaporation	Body heat is used to evaporate liquid on the skin.	Sweating is how your body tries to keep cool on a hot day.	Keep your skin as dry as possible.
4. Conduction	Heat moves directly from the body to a cold object that the body is touching.	Sitting on the cold ground or wearing wet clothing—your heat moves from you into the ground or wet clothing.	Don't get wet. Wear fabric next to your skin that moves the wet away (e.g. polypropylene).
5. Convection (wind chill)	The thin layer of warm air around the body is replaced by cooler air, which the body must now heat.	The wind blows through openings in your clothing and blows the warm air against your skin away.	Wear windproof clothing with snug cuffs and collars to keep the wind out.

Hypothermia

The normal temperature of the body's core is 37° C (98.6° F). If the body core temperature drops more than two degrees, the body's tissues cannot function properly. This state of generalized cooling is called hypothermia. Hypothermia, often called exposure, kills many Canadians each year—but it is a condition that can be detected and corrected by a first aider if recognized early.

Who gets hypothermia?

Anyone can become hypothermic, but the following groups are especially prone:

◆ elderly people, because they often have poor circulation, less ability to sense the cold, and may be on medication that promotes heat loss

◆ babies have less ability to recover from mild and moderate hypothermia because they lose heat more quickly and their bodies don't control body heat as well

◆ people who are already weakened due to illness, injury, lack of food, fatigue or through the use of alcohol or drugs

◆ teenagers, because they often underdress for the weather conditions

Signs of hypothermia			
Sign	Mild	Moderate	Severe
pulse	normal	slow and weak	weak, irregular or absent
breathing	normal	slow and shallow	slow or absent
appearance	shivering, slurred speech	shivering violently , clumsy, stumbling, pupils dilated, skin bluish	shivering has stopped
mental state	conscious but withdrawn or disinterested	confused, sleepy irrational	unconscious

Signs of hypothermia

There are three stages of hypothermia: mild, moderate and severe. The table on page 300 lists the signs for each stage, but it may be hard to tell exactly when one stage ends and another begins. Body temperatures are not listed here because the first aider has no practical way to take the temperature of the body's core.

Recognizing hypothermia

The key to successful first aid for hypothermia is recognizing the casualty's condition as soon as possible, and preventing hypothermia from getting worse. Hypothermia is the obvious thing to look for on a cold winter day, but it is less obvious when the temperature is above zero. Be on the lookout for hypothermia whenever the temperature is below 20° C, the weather is windy, wet or both, or the casualty is in one of the groups at risk for hypothermia.

Sometimes hypothermia is mistaken for other conditions. Hypothermia has been mistaken for drunkenness, stroke and drug abuse. This often happens in the city, where a warm environment doesn't seem far away. For example, an elderly person's home may not feel cold to you since you are warmly dressed, but in fact the room temperature is 15° C, the elderly person is underdressed, and is hypothermic.

And don't forget yourself—as soon as you begin to shiver, think "I've got to prevent further heat loss." If you don't, hypothermia will soon affect your mind, and you won't be able to think clearly enough to take the right actions.

First aid for hypothermia

First aid for hypothermia aims to prevent further heat loss and get medical help.

1   Begin ESM—do a scene survey. If the temperature is lower than 20° C, suspect hypothermia either as the casualty's main problem or as a complication of another injury.

2   Do a primary survey and take measures to prevent further heat loss:

◆   cover exposed skin with suitable clothing or covers; make sure the head is well insulated

◆   adjust the casualty's clothing to keep wind or drafts out. Wrap the casualty in something windproof—reflective "space blankets" and plastic garbage bags are good for this

◆   if possible, move the casualty out of the cold environment. If you cannot move indoors, protect the casualty from the wind

◆   loosen or remove tight clothing

◆   wet clothing causes severe heat loss. If you are in a shelter and have a dry change of clothes, gently replace wet clothes with dry ones. If you are not sheltered, put the dry clothes over the wet clothes. If you don't have dry clothes, press as much water out of the wet clothes as possible and wrap the casualty with something windproof

◆   insulate the casualty from cold objects—have him sit on a rolled-up jacket or lie on a blanket

◆   get medical help. If you have to arrange transportation, the casualty should be moved in

the recovery position

3 Give ongoing casualty care, monitoring the ABCs. If the casualty is not breathing begin CPR, but do not delay transporting the casualty.

Immersion hypothermia

Immersion hypothermia refers to hypothermia caused by being in cold water. A person loses heat 25–30 times faster in water than in air of the same temperature. Immersion hypothermia can happen very quickly, within minutes, if a person falls into cold water. Suspect hypothermia whenever someone falls into water by mistake even in the summer. Immersion hypothermia can also happen more slowly, for instance while swimming or scuba diving in a lake. In these cases, hypothermia creeps up on the casualty, and may not be suspected right away.

Do the following when a hypothermic casualty is in the water:

◆ tell the casualty not to take off any clothing—clothing helps keep heat in

◆ tell the casualty to move as little as possible—moving around causes more heat loss (by convection)

When taking a casualty out of the water, keep him in a horizontal position, and handle him as gently as possible. Give first aid for hypothermia as outlined on page 302, to prevent further heat loss, and get medical help.

If you are the casualty, use the "heat escape lessening position" (HELP) to preserve body heat until help arrives.

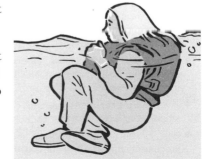

Frostbite

Frostbite refers to the freezing of tissues when exposed to temperatures below zero. It is a progressive injury with two stages: superficial frostbite and deep frostbite.

 First aid for superficial frostbite

1   Begin ESM—do a scene survey. Gradually rewarm the frostbitten part with body heat .

♦ cover frostbitten toes, ears, etc. with warm hands

♦ warm up frostbitten fingers by breathing on them or placing them in a warm area of the body like the armpit, abdomen or groin

2   Take measures to prevent these areas from freezing again—either stop the activity or dress more appropriately.

Cautions in first aid for hypothermia

♦ Handle the casualty very gently and keep him horizontal if possible. Cold affects the electrical impulses that make the heart beat. As a result, the hypothermic casualty's heart beat is very delicate. The heart can stop with rough handling of the casualty.

♦ If trained to check for a pulse in a casualty who may be hypothermic, continue checking for 30 to 45 seconds. The heart may be beating slowly or very faintly and it may take longer to find the pulse.

♦ Don't give the casualty any alcohol, coffee, or other drinks with caffeine, or let him smoke —these can increase heat loss.

♦ Don't rub the casualty's body to improve circulation—this will cause cold blood to flow back to the body core and cool the body further.

First aid for deep frostbite

How much tissue is permanently damaged by deep frostbite depends on how long the part was frozen, how much the part was used while frozen and how the part was thawed. Deep frostbite needs medical help as soon as possible.

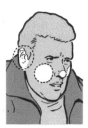

frostbitten skin looks white and waxy

1   Begin ESM—do a scene survey. Prevent further heat loss from the frozen part and the rest of the body. Handle the frozen tissue very gently to prevent further tissue damage.

Do not rub the arms and legs. Keep the casualty as still as possible.

2   Get medical help. If the feet or legs are frozen, don't let the casualty walk (if possible)—transport using a rescue carry or stretcher (see page 79).

If medical help is not available, you are in a safe, warm place and there is no danger of the part refreezing, then thaw the frozen part according to the instructions on the next page.

7

Stages of frostbite and their signs and symptoms

Stage	Description		Signs & symptoms
superficial frostbite	The full thickness of the skin is frozen.		– white, waxy-looking skin – skin is firm to touch, but tissue underneath is soft – may feel pain at first, followed by numbness
deep frostbite	The skin, and the tissues underneath the skin, are frozen, sometimes to the bone. A serious condition, often involving an entire hand or foot.		– white, waxy-looking skin that turns greyish-blue as frostbite progresses – skin feels cold and hard – there is no feeling in the area

◆ Make the casualty warm and as comfortable as possible. Gently remove the clothing from the affected part. Find a container that is large enough to hold the entire frozen part. Fill this with water that feels warm when you put your elbow in it (about 40° C). Make sure you have more water at this temperature available.

◆ Remove any jewellery and put the whole frozen part in the water. Keep adding warm water to keep the water in the container at a constant temperature. Keep the part in the water until it is pink or does not improve any more—this can take up to 40 minutes, and may be painful.

◆ Gently dry the affected part. Put sterile dressings over wounds and between fingers or toes.

◆ Keep the part elevated and warm. Do not break any blisters that form.

8 Give ongoing casualty care.

If the casualty must walk, do not thaw the frozen part—there will be less tissue damage and pain if the part is left frozen. Make sure the rest of the body is well protected from the cold and the casualty has plenty of food and water during the journey to safety.

Frozen state

When the temperature is below zero, it is possible to discover someone who is completely frozen—this is a frozen state. Recognize a frozen state when:

◆ the casualty is found in a cold location and is unresponsive

◆ the joints of the jaw and neck are rigid when you try to open the airway

- the skin and deeper tissues are cold and cannot be depressed

- the entire body moves as a solid unit

If the casualty is in a frozen state, do not attempt first aid for the ABCs. Transport the casualty to medical help if this doesn't pose a risk to the rescuers. Otherwise, get yourself to safety and advise the police of the location of the frozen person.

Cautions in first aid for frostbite

- Do not rub the area—the tiny ice crystals in the tissues may cause more tissue damage.

- Do not rub snow on the area—this may cause further freezing and tissue damage from the rubbing.

- Do not apply direct heat; this may rewarm the area too quickly.

7

Rewarming a casualty

Types of rewarming

There are two types of rewarming: passive rewarming and active rewarming. Passive rewarming means preventing further heat loss and letting the casualty's body rewarm itself—this usually works well for mild and moderate hypothermia. Active rewarming means adding heat to the casualty's body to warm it up. Active rewarming can cause complications and should only be done at a hospital—but active rewarming is what a casualty in severe hypothermia needs. This is why in severe hypothermia the first aid is to prevent further heat loss and safely transport the casualty to medical help.

Active rewarming by the first aider

In mild hypothermia, you can give the fully conscious casualty something warm and sweet to drink. The sweetened drink will provide energy to the muscles and help the body to continue shivering. Don't give a casualty in moderate hypothermia anything to drink. His muscles for swallowing may not work well and he could choke. Only if you are far from medical aid should you actively rewarm a casualty. Do this by placing the casualty near a heat source and placing containers of warm, but not hot, water in contact with the skin (neck, armpits, groin). Prevent further heat loss and get medical help as soon as possible.

Heat exposure and illnesses

Prolonged exposure to extreme heat or heavy exertion in a hot environment can cause heat illnesses.

Heat cramps

Heat cramps are painful muscle cramps, usually in the legs and abdomen, caused by losing too much water and salt through sweating. Heat cramps are usually caused by heavy exercise or physical work in a hot environment. They are not serious and may be reversed by first aid. The casualty will complain of cramps and show signs of excessive sweating.

In a dry environment, the casualty may not seem to be sweating because the sweat evaporates quickly.

First aid for heat cramps

1   Begin ESM—do a scene survey. Place the casualty at rest in a cool place.

2   Give the conscious casualty water or drinks with electrolytes and carbohydrates. She can have as much as she wants.

3   If the cramps don't go away, get medical help.

Heat exhaustion

Heat exhaustion is more serious than heat cramps. The casualty has lost fluid through sweating. Circulation is affected because the blood flows away from the major organs and pools in the blood vessels just below the skin.

Signs and symptoms of heat exhaustion

◆ excessive sweating and dilated pupils

◆ casualty may complain of dizziness, blurred vision, headache or cramps

◆ signs of shock, including: cold, clammy skin; weak, rapid pulse; rapid, shallow breathing; vomiting and unconsciousness

 ### First aid for heat exhaustion

First aid for heat exhaustion combines the first aid for heat cramps with the first aid for shock.

1   Begin ESM—do a scene survey and a primary survey. Send for medical help.

2   If the casualty is conscious:

◆ give the conscious casualty water or drinks with electro-lytes and carbohydrates. If the casualty vomits, don't give anything by mouth and get medical help right away

◆ place her at rest on her back in a cool place

◆ remove excessive clothing and loosen tight clothing at the neck and waist

If the casualty is unconscious:

◆ place her in the recovery position

◆ get medical help right away

◆ monitor ABCs and give life-saving first aid as needed

7

3   Give ongoing casualty care until medical help takes over

Heatstroke (sunstroke)

Heatstroke is a life-threatening condition where the body's temperature rises far above normal. It is caused by prolonged exposure in a hot, humid, and perhaps poorly ventilated environment. In classic heatstroke, the body's temperature control mechanism fails, sweating stops and the body temperature rises rapidly. In exertional heatstroke, the body temperature rises rapidly due to heavy physical exertion in high temperatures, even though sweating continues. Elderly people and those in poor health are more likely to suffer from heatstroke. Without immediate first aid heatstroke can result in permanent brain damage or death .

Signs and symptoms of heatstroke

◆ body temperature rapidly rises to 40°C or higher—the casualty is hot to the touch

◆ the pulse is rapid and full but gets weaker in later stages

◆ breathing is noisy

◆ skin is flushed, hot and dry in classic heatstroke, and flushed, hot and sweaty in exertional heatstroke

◆ casualty is restless and may complain of headache, fatigue, dizziness and nausea

◆ vomiting, convulsions, unconsciousness

You can tell the difference between heat exhaustion and heatstroke by the condition of the skin. In heat exhaustion, the skin is moist and cold. In heatstroke, the skin is hot, flushed and may be dry or wet.

First aid for heatstroke

1   Begin ESM—do a scene survey. Lowering body temperature is the most urgent first aid for heatstroke. The casualty's life depends on how quickly this can be done.

◆ move the casualty to a cool, shaded place

◆ cool the casualty—remove outer clothing and immerse the casualty in cold water up to the chin—watch her closely

If this is not possible:

❖ cover her with wet sheets and fan the sheets to increase cooling

❖ sponge the casualty with cool water, particularly in the armpits, neck and groin areas

2   When her body feels cool to touch, cover her with a dry sheet. Put the conscious casualty into the shock position and the unconscious casualty into the recovery position. Monitor the casualty closely. If her temperature begins to rise again, repeat the cooling process.

3   Give ongoing casualty care until handover to medical help.

7

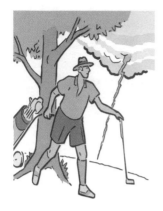

Lightning injuries

Electrical storms occur throughout most of Canada. Although people generally think that the chance of being struck by lightning is very low, there are many injuries and deaths each year from lightning strikes.

Give first aid at the scene of a lightning strike as you would any other emergency scene, keeping the following in mind:

◆ a person struck by lightning does not hold an electrical charge. In a lightning strike, the lightning often travels around the person rather than through him—you can touch the casualty without fear of electric shock

7

◆ the casualty has probably been thrown—suspect a head or spinal injury

◆ lightning does strike the same place twice—assess the risk of another strike, and move to a safer location if needed

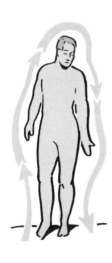

◆ if more than one person is injured, the principles of multiple casualty management are reversed—give first aid to unresponsive non-breathing casualties since the casualties still breathing are on the road to recovery

◆ advise all casualties of a lightning strike to seek medical help to ensure a full evaluation of any injuries

Poisoning

A poison is any substance that can cause illness or death when absorbed by the body. There are poisonous substances all around us. Poisonous consumer products have poison symbols on their labels, but there are many other poisonous substances that don't carry warnings. Examples include alcohol, some common household plants, contaminated food, and medications when not taken as prescribed. Many substances that are not harmful in small amounts may be poisonous in large amounts.

poison symbol

Types of poisons

Poisons are classified according to how they enter the body:

◆ swallowed poisons—through the mouth

◆ inhaled poisons—through the lungs

◆ absorbed poisons—through the skin and mucous membranes

◆ injected poisons—through a hollow needle or needle-like device (e.g. a snake's fangs)

An important part of the first aid for poisoning is telephoning the Poison Information Centre for advice on what to do. Before calling, the first aider must quickly gather as much information about the incident as possible. Use the history of the scene and the signs and symptoms of the casualty to gather the information you'll need to answer the questions asked by the Poison Information Centre.

History of the scene

Poisoning may occur despite all reasonable precautions. When it does, act quickly but do not panic. You need to know four basic facts to give appropriate first aid for poisoning:

◆ what poison was taken—container labels should identify the poison; otherwise, save vomit and give it to medical help for analysis

◆ how much poison was taken—estimate the quantity that may have been taken based on what you see or are told—the number of pills originally in the container, the amount of chemical in the bottle, etc. Estimate the size/age of the casualty

◆ how the poison entered the body—first aid may differ for poisons taken by mouth, absorbed through the skin, injected into the blood or breathed into the lungs

◆ when the poison was taken—the length of time the poison has been in the body will help determine the first aid and medical care needed

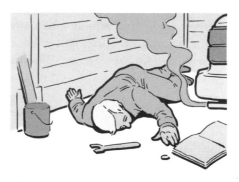

Signs and symptoms of poisoning

If the history does not reveal what poison was taken, or by what means it was taken, signs and symptoms may be helpful in answering these questions. All poisons may affect consciousness, breathing and pulse. Other signs and symptoms may vary depending on how the poison was taken. Poisons that have been:

◆ swallowed usually cause nausea, abdominal cramps, diarrhea and vomiting. They may discolour the lips, cause burns in or around the mouth or leave an odour on the breath

◆ absorbed through the skin may cause a reddening of the skin, blisters, swelling and burns

◆ injected through the skin usually irritate the point of entry

◆ inhaled may cause problems with breathing.

Signs and symptoms may include coughing, chest pain and difficulty breathing. Prolonged exposure to natural gas used for heating or carbon monoxide (CO) from combustion engines will cause headache, dizziness, unconsciousness, stopped breathing and cardiac arrest.

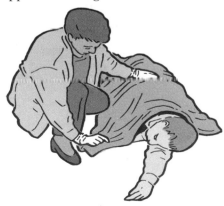

General first aid for poisoning

1   Begin ESM—do a scene survey. Gather any information about the suspected poison. Assess the casualty's responsiveness.

   ◆ if the casualty is responsive, call the Poison Information Centre in your region, or your hospital emergency department. Answer any questions and follow their advice on first aid

   ◆ if the casualty is unresponsive, call medical help (e.g. an ambulance) immediately and go to step 2

2   Do a primary survey. If breathing is stopped begin CPR. Check for poisonous material around the mouth first. Use a barrier device if you have one.

3   Place the unconscious breathing casualty into the recovery position.

4   Give ongoing casualty care until medical help takes over.

7

Poison Information Centre

The phone number for your local Poison Information Centre is listed at the beginning of your telephone directory.

First aid for swallowed poisons

1 Begin ESM—do a scene survey and a primary survey.

2 Do not dilute a poison that has been swallowed (do not give fluids) unless told to do so by the Poison Information Centre.

3 If the casualty is conscious, wipe poisonous or corrosive residue from the casualty's face and rinse or wipe out the mouth.

4 Never induce vomiting except on the advice of the Poison Information Centre—many poisons will cause more damage when vomited.

First aid for inhaled poisons

1 Begin ESM—do a scene survey. Assess hazards with particular attention to the possible presence of a poisonous gas or vapour.   Ensure your safety; it may be best to wait for professional rescuers.

2 Inhaled poisons, such as gases, should be cleared from the lungs as quickly as possible. Move the person to fresh air and away from the source of the poison.

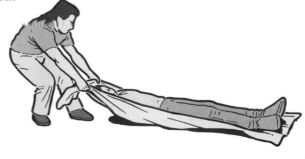

3 If the casualty is unresponsive, call for medical help right away.

4 Do a primary survey and give first aid for the ABCs. If breathing is not present begin CPR. If the poison could affect you while giving first aid, use a face mask or shield with a one-way valve.

5 If the casualty vomits, keep the airway open by clearing out the mouth and putting the casualty into the recovery position.

6 If the casualty goes into convulsions, prevent him from injuring himself.

7 Get medical help. Give ongoing casualty care, monitoring the casualty closely.

 First aid for absorbed poisons

Most poisons absorbed by the skin cause irritation at the place of contact, but don't affect the rest of the body. The irritation, called contact dermatitis, includes redness, itching and blisters.

Some chemicals, however, do affect the rest of the body when absorbed by the skin, and these can cause life-threatening emergencies.

1 Begin ESM—do a scene survey.

2 Do a primary survey and give first aid for life-threatening conditions.

3 Flush the affected area with large amounts of cool water.

◆ if the poisonous substance is a powder, brush off excessive amounts with a dry cloth before flushing

4 Remove any clothing that has been in contact with the poison. Don't touch the clothing until it has been thoroughly washed. Try not to touch the affected part of the body to any other part of the body.

5 Wash the affected skin thoroughly with soap and water.

◆ pay careful attention to hidden areas such as under the fingernails and in the hair

6 Give ongoing casualty care until medical help takes over.

 First aid for injected poisons

Follow the general first aid for poisoning (see page 316). Injected poisons should be contained near the injection site. Delay the circulation of the poison through out the body by placing the casualty at rest and keeping the affected limb below heart level.

If you have been pricked with a needle with possible HIV or other transmissable disease contamination, then the site of the needlestick injury should be vigorously scrubbed with Iodine or similar disinfectant. Get medical attention.

Emergency Childbirth and Miscarriage

Emergency childbirth occurs when a child is born at an unplanned time or at an unplanned place. This may happen when there is a sudden, premature delivery or when the mother cannot get to the hospital for a full-term delivery. Miscarriage, also called spontaneous abortion, occurs when the fetus is "born" before it is developed enough to survive. This is before the 20th week of pregnancy.

Anatomy

A basic knowledge of the female reproductive system during pregnancy will help you to give the needed care and protection during an emergency delivery.

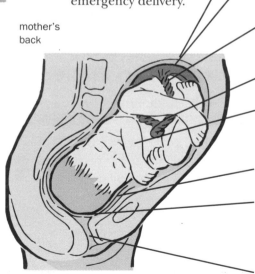

mother's back

uterus—the hollow, muscular structure, also called the womb, that holds the developing baby

placenta—a large, flat, spongy organ that is attached to the inside wall of the uterus, that supplies the fetus with nutrients and oxygen from the mother

umbilical cord—a rope-like structure that carries blood between the mother and the fetus

fetus—what the baby is called until it is born

amniotic sac—the bag that the fetus develops in; it is full of fluid called amniotic fluid

amniotic fluid—liquid that surrounds and protects the fetus in the amniotic sac

cervix—the neck of the uterus that opens during labour so the fetus can be born

vagina—the muscular passageway through which the baby is born, also called the birth canal

7

Pregnancy and childbirth

A normal pregnancy is 40 weeks. If the baby is born before the 37th week, it is considered premature. If the baby is born between the 37th and 42nd week, it is full term. Most babies born are full term, but it is not uncommon for a baby to be born prematurely.

A baby is born in a three-stage process called labour. It can be hard to tell when labour has started, but it has probably begun when one of the following happens:

◆ the uterus contracts at regular intervals of ten to twenty minutes, with contractions getting increasingly stronger and closer together

◆ amniotic fluid comes out of the vagina, which means the amniotic sac has broken—this may be called the "water breaking." There may be a trickle or a rush of fluid

◆ blood and mucus come from the vagina—this "bloody show" means that the mucus plug that had sealed the cervix has come out because the cervix has started to open

Stage 1: Early labour—opening of the cervix

The first stage of labour, called early labour, can take up to eighteen hours for a first child, but may be much shorter for the second or subsequent children. Usually there is enough time to get the mother to a medical facility. Early labour involves muscular contractions that may begin as an aching feeling in the lower back. As contractions get stronger, they feel like cramps in the lower abdomen. Contractions cause the cervix to open, or dilate. The cervix has to dilate until the opening is about 10 cm across before the fetus can be pushed down the birth canal, which is the second stage of labour.

Stage 2: Birth of the baby

The second stage of labour usually takes about one hour. It begins when the cervix is fully dilated and the contractions start to push the fetus out of the uterus and through the vagina. When the baby's head is close to the vaginal opening, the mother may feel a tremendous urge to push the fetus out. Usually, the fetus' head is born first, then one shoulder, then the other shoulder, and then the rest of the body is pushed out quite quickly. The second stage of labour ends when the baby is born. The baby is still connected to the mother by the umbilical cord. The cord is attached to the placenta, still in the uterus.

Stage 3: Delivery of the placenta

The third stage of labour is the delivery of the placenta after the baby is born. The uterus gets smaller and pushes the placenta out. This stage usually takes ten to twenty minutes. Labour is finished when the placenta is delivered.

Emergency childbirth

Your role as a first aider in emergency childbirth is to help the mother deliver the baby, to protect the mother and baby, and to save all parts of the placenta and amniotic sac until medical help takes over.

Assessing the stage of labour

If the mother is still in early labour, you probably still have time to get her to a hospital—if you are not sure, call for medical help and stay where you are. If labour is in the second stage, the baby will be born quite soon. Recognize the second stage of labour by:

♦ longer and stronger contractions, less than two minutes apart

◆ the mother's previous experience—if she says the baby is coming, believe her

◆ bulging of the vaginal opening and seeing the baby's head (called crowning)

◆ the mother is straining and pushing down, and feels like she has to have a bowel movement

When you see these signs, you will not have time to get the mother to medical help. Call medical help to the scene, if possible, and get ready to deliver the baby.

 Emergency delivery

1   Begin ESM—do the scene survey. Locate someone to help you, preferably a female. Get the materials you will need to deliver the baby and the placenta. You may find some of these things in a bag the mother has packed for the hospital.

2   During early labour, let the mother find the position of most comfort—usually on her left side. Put a folded towel under her right hip if she wants to lie on her back.

Encourage the mother to empty her bladder and bowels as often as possible to avoid complications later. It is also important at this stage that the mother does not push or strain with the contractions. She should try to breathe and relax through them.

3   During the second stage of labour, when the baby will be born very soon, place the mother on her back with knees bent and head supported, unless she

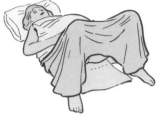

prefers another position. Cover her with sheets so you can easily lift them to check on the progress of labour.

Reassure the mother and try to appear calm and unhurried. When the mother is in position, put on your gloves, or wash your hands, arms and fingernails.

4 Tell your assistant to help the mother through the contractions. When you can see the baby's head, the mother can push with the contractions. Tell her to wait until the contraction peaks, then take a deep breath, put her chin on her chest and push down as hard and as long as she can, while she is holding her breath. She may be able to push like this twice for each contraction. Position yourself to watch for the baby.

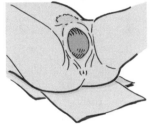

5 When you see the baby, get ready to deliver it. Usually the head is born first and if it comes out too quickly, the baby could be injured. As the head comes out, tell the mother to control her pushing. One way for her to do this is to breathe in fast, shallow breaths (panting).

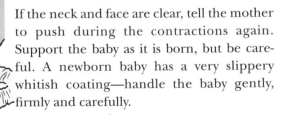

If the neck and face are clear, tell the mother to push during the contractions again. Support the baby as it is born, but be careful. A newborn baby has a very slippery whitish coating—handle the baby gently, firmly and carefully.

6 Clear the baby's airway—all babies have fluid in the nose and throat. Hold the baby with the head lower than the body to help drainage.

7 Most babies will cry right away. When they do, they become pink as they start breathing. If the baby doesn't start to breathe and remains pale and limp, try stimulating him. If the baby still doesn't breathe, start infant CPR (see page 141).

8 Once the baby is breathing, pat him dry with a towel, being careful not to remove the slippery coating. Wrap the baby in a dry towel or blanket to keep him warm. Check the umbilical cord. If the cord is still pulsating, keep the baby at the level of the vagina. If the cord has stopped pulsating, place the baby on his side in the mother's arms with his head low to assist drainage. The baby may want to nurse at the mother's breast.

9 Check the vagina for bleeding. If bleeding from the vagina is severe—act quickly. The umbilical cord must be tied because the baby's blood may be bleeding through the cord and out of the placenta. Tie the umbilical cord and keep the baby at the same level as the vagina.

10 Wait for the placenta to be delivered. This usually happens within twenty minutes of the baby's birth, but don't be surprised if it takes longer. Gently massaging the mother's lower abdomen will quicken the delivery of the placenta.

11 There may be some bleeding from the vagina after the delivery of the placenta. This is normal, and can usually be controlled by firmly massaging the uterus. The uterus can be felt as a hard, round mass in the lower abdomen. Massaging it every few minutes will help it to contract which helps control any bleeding. The baby's nursing at the mother's breast also helps to contract the uterus. Use sanitary pads to absorb any bleeding. If the bleeding cannot be controlled, transport to medical help as soon as possible.

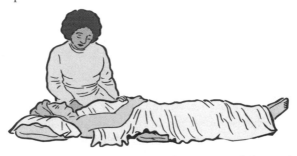

Examine the skin between the anus and the vagina for lacerations and apply pressure with sterile dressings to any bleeding tears of the skin.

12 Give ongoing casualty care to the mother and infant. Keep them warm and comfortable and transport them to medical help as soon as possible.

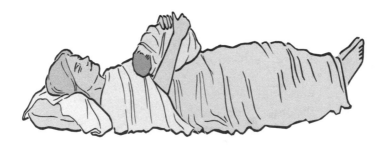

Vaginal bleeding and miscarriage

Miscarriage is the loss of the fetus before the 20th week of pregnancy. Most miscarriages happen because the fetus was not developing properly and was not able to survive. The medical term for a miscarriage is spontaneous abortion.

Signs and symptoms

◆ vaginal bleeding that could be severe

◆ signs of shock

◆ cramp-like pains in the lower abdomen

◆ aching in the lower back

◆ passage of tissue

 First aid for miscarriage

Your main concern in first aid for miscarriage is shock caused by severe bleeding. The woman may be very distressed.

1   Begin ESM—do a scene survey.

2   Do a primary survey. Give first aid for shock—place the woman on her back, or on her left side. Call for medical help immediately.

Ensure privacy. Reassure her and give her emotional support. If the woman is upset over losing the baby, explain that the miscarriage was not her fault and was not caused by anything she did.

Keep any evidence of tissue and blood loss (bloody sheets, clothing, etc.). Send this with the woman to medical help for examination by the doctor.

3   Give ongoing casualty care.

Psychological Emergencies

A psychological emergency occurs when a person's state of mind makes it difficult for her to cope with the situation at hand. Your role as a first aider is to help the casualty cope, while protecting her, and others at the scene, until medical help arrives.

There are many causes of psychological emergencies. Knowing the cause of a person's behaviour helps you to decide the best first aid. Some psychological emergencies you may encounter include:

◆ hysteria

◆ anxiety and panic attacks

◆ emotional reaction to assault

◆ alcohol and drug-induced behaviour

◆ mental illness and suicide gestures

General first aid for psychological emergencies

1 Begin ESM—do a scene survey. In a psychological emergency:

◆ always approach the casualty from the front

◆ identify yourself as a first aider and offer to help. The casualty may refuse your help. If you suspect the casualty isn't able to make a responsible decision about needing help, consider helping anyway

2 Do a primary survey and give first aid for life-threatening emergencies—these are always the priority.

Note the casualty's vital signs. Be alert to any changes in the casualty's condition since there may be "unseen" reasons for the behavioural emergency like a head injury or medical condition.

3 Find out the history of the emergency by questioning the casualty and others at the scene. It may take some time before the casualty will talk about the situation.

4 Provide quiet, supportive, reassuring care while arranging for medical help. If the casualty shows any signs of aggressive behaviour, or if you think a crime has taken place, call the police to the scene.

Give first aid for a psychological emergency in a warm, sensitive and compassionate manner. Remember to:

◆ control your own emotions at the scene. Don't overreact to the casualty's behaviour or to emotional attacks directed at you

◆ only get involved to the level you feel comfortable— don't put yourself at risk

◆ only make promises you can keep, and don't lie to the person in any way

◆ include the casualty's friends and/or family in giving care—these people may be able to reassure and help the casualty

◆ be careful whenever there is aggressive behaviour—avoid restraining the casualty—only use restraint to ensure the safety of others

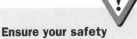

Ensure your safety

If the casualty is violent, or you think she may become violent, keep your distance and be very careful. Don't stop the casualty from leaving the area—especially don't block the casualty's exit. Let the casualty go and call the police.

Anxiety (panic) attack

During an anxiety attack, the casualty shows the normal response of a person faced with a life-threatening situation, but there is no threatening situation at hand. Anxiety attacks are quite common.

Signs and symptoms of an anxiety attack

◆ a feeling of fear or a sense that something terrible will happen

◆ the casualty may say:

❖ "I can feel my heart pounding!"

❖ "I feel like I'm smothering. . . I just can't get enough air!"

❖ "I'm having trouble swallowing."

◆ trembling and sweating

◆ hyperventilation, tingling hands and feet

◆ nausea or vomiting

 First aid for an anxiety attack

1   Give the same first aid as for hysteria —see previous page.

2   If the casualty is hyperventilating, give first aid for hyperventilation (see page 110).

3   Give first aid for any signs and symptoms.

4   Get medical help. Stay with the casualty until medical help takes over.

Hysteria (conversion disorder)

Hysteria is a psychological emergency that causes violent fits of laughing and/or crying, imagined illnesses and a general lack of self-control.

Signs and symptoms of hysteria

◆ loss of control of behaviour that may show as shouting, rolling on the ground, and beating the chest. Behaviour is often made worse by the presence of an audience

◆ hyperventilation that may be severe, causing muscle spasms, especially in the wrists and hands

◆ obvious tremors or "paralysis." The casualty is apparently unable to move.

 First aid for hysteria

1 Begin ESM—do a scene survey and a primary survey.

2 Lead the casualty to a quiet place, away from onlookers, and try to help the casualty calm down and regain self-control.

3 Be firm and positive. Do not over-sympathize. Listen calmly as the casualty talks. Do not question or contradict the casualty.

4 It may help to "give the casualty permission" to start feeling better. A hysterical casualty may be very "suggestible" this way. For example, say, "I see your legs aren't working now, but I'm sure they will feel better in a couple of minutes."

5 Stay with the casualty until medical help takes over.

Physical and sexual assault

Being assaulted is a devastating life crisis because it involves both emotional and physical violence. Along with physical injuries, sexual assault casualties often go into severe emotional shock during or shortly after the attack. Signs and symptoms of this emotional state include:

◆ choking, gagging, nausea, vomiting

◆ hyperventilation

◆ casualty seems dazed

◆ seizures or loss of consciousness

 General first aid for assault

1 Begin ESM—do a scene survey. If you suspect an assault, don't disturb evidence by removing, washing, or disposing of clothing.

2 Do a primary survey. Give first aid for life-threatening injuries.

3 Give general first aid for psychological emergencies (see page 328). Tell the casualty not to wash, and if possible, not to use the toilet until told to do so by a trained health professional.

Drugs, including alcohol

Drugs are defined as any substance that can produce a physical or mental effect on the body. They include alcohol, prescription drugs and illegal substances. The effects of drugs are wide-ranging and can be unpredictable. Dosages and combinations of drugs (including alcohol) will affect the casualty's condition. Be prepared for behaviour which can change quickly.

First aid for a casualty on drugs or alcohol

1   Begin ESM—do a scene survey. Approach the casualty in a calm, professional, sympathetic manner and try to gain her confidence.

Be aware of the possibility of infectious hepatitis or AIDS caused by using contaminated needles—use personal protective equipment (PPE) to avoid infection (see page 17).

Try to find out the type and amount of the drug consumed.

2   Perform a primary survey. Monitor the ABCs frequently. If the casualty has convulsions, vomiting or unconsciousness, be sure to maintain an open airway and effective breathing.

Check for possible fractures or other injuries and give appropriate first aid. Do not leave the casualty.

3   Give ongoing casualty care as appropriate and get medical help.

7

Mental illness and suicidal gestures

When there are no other obvious causes, you can assume that persistent abnormal behaviour results from some form of mental illness. Give general first aid for psychological emergencies and get medical help.

Any threats of suicide must be taken very seriously. A person who threatens to commit suicide is usually severely disturbed and suffers some underlying emotional illness. Give the first aid required for any injuries. Use a calm, professional approach at all times and work to establish trust and confidence. Never lie to the casualty. Do not leave the casualty alone. Keep the casualty from harm by whatever means possible.

Call the police and give ongoing casualty care until help arrives.

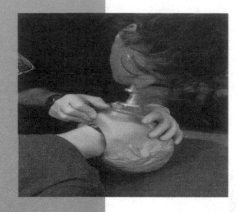

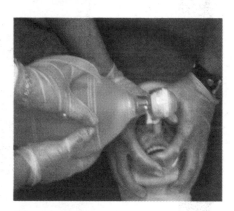

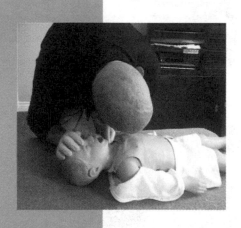

8

RESUSCITATION SKILLS FOR HEALTH CARE PROVIDERS

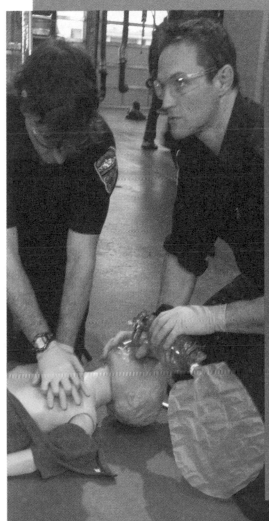

- ♦ *An introduction to advanced techniques*

- ♦ *Artificial respiration*

- ♦ *Assisted breathing*

- ♦ *Using a bag-valve mask (BVM)*

- ♦ *Variations on CPR techniques*

- ♦ *Two rescuer CPR*

- ♦ *AED*

Introduction

This chapter presents information and skills that will be relevant to the health care provider. Health care providers include a variety of professionals who may or may not, hold licenses or certifications. Health care providers in Canada may include medical and nursing students, physicians, nurses, paramedics, respiratory therapists, physical and occupational therapists, other allied health personnel, industrial emergency response teams as well as volunteer and career firefighters. Professionals with a duty to respond—who are specifically responsible for responding to, or providing care will take specific training before they are authorized to use these skills.

CPR is only effective if there is adequate coronary and cerebral circulation. Improper compressions and ventilations can have a negative impact on patient outcome. Interruptions in compressions will decrease the all important coronary and cerebral circulation. While excessive ventilations will increase the pressure inside the chest, the amount of blood returning to the heart decreases. This in turn diminishes the amount of blood that can be circulated from the heart and decreases the chances of survival.

In the case of sudden cardiac arrest, every minute after collapse, without CPR, reduces the chances of survival by 7 to 10% per minute from time of collapse. However, when high quality CPR and defibrillation is provided from the onset of collapse the chances of survival improve. High quality CPR includes uninterrupted compression rate of at least 100 per minute, appropriate compression depth based on the age of the casualty and allowing for complete chest recoil after each compression.

There are a number of differences in how the health care provider is expected to respond to an emergency. Based on their level of training, health care providers are encouraged to tailor rescue actions to the most likely cause of arrest.

It is important to remember that where local protocols (including legislation, medical direction and professional/ workplace requirements) differ from this information, the local protocol supercedes information in this chapter.

Age Categories for CPR

The health care provider will respond to casualties based on the following categories:

Adult—onset of puberty and older

Child—1 year of age to the onset of puberty (about 12 to 14 years, as defined by the presence of secondary sex characteristics)

Infant—anyone under the age of 1 year

Neonate/newborn—an infant who has been delivered, and in the first hours after birth and until they leave the hospital. The health care provider will not need to differentiate this group from other infants, unless they are specifically trained to provide resuscitative care for that age group.

8

Activation of Emergency Medical Response System

Health care providers should be familiar with when and how to activate their own internal and/or external Emergency Medical Response system. A plan should be in place to allow for an AED to arrive on scene with the rescuer or for an AED to be quickly retrieved and easily accessible. Casualty outcomes will be improved by having rapid access to CPR, AED and Advanced Life Support. The following information provides guidelines on how to initially respond to a casualty:

Casualties of all ages—2 Rescuers

Anytime two rescuers are present, one rescuer will stay and begin CPR while the second rescuer will activate the Emergency Medical Response System and obtain an AED, if one is not already present.

Adult Casualty—Lone Rescuer

The section on Medical Help in Chapter 1 of this reference guide will help you decide when you should leave a casualty to go for help. Remember that anyone in cardiac arrest will need CPR, defibrillation and Advanced Life Support.

The lone rescuer who encounters a witnessed arrest or an unwitnessed unresponsive adult casualty should activate the Emergency Medical Response System immediately.

When a casualty of any age is believed to have suffered an asphyxial (lack of oxygen) arrest, the lone rescuer should provide two minutes of CPR before activating the Emergency Medical Response System and obtaining the AED. This is done because the casualty has been deprived of oxygen, resulting in the arrest. The objective is to correct the cause of the arrest. By performing two minutes of CPR first, the rescuer is taking the initial steps to correct the cause of the arrest.

Child Casualty—Lone Rescuer

When the lone rescuer witnesses a child casualty suddenly collapse they should immediately activate their Emergency Medical Response System and obtain and use the AED right away.

The lone rescuer who does not witness the arrest should provide two minutes of CPR before activating the Emergency Medical Response System.

When activating the Emergency Medical Response System, the rescuer may consider carrying the child if the child is small enough, if injuries permit and if the distance they must go does not impact on the start or resumption of CPR.

Infant Casualty—Lone Rescuer

When the lone rescuer witnesses an infant casualty suddenly collapse, they should activate the Emergency Medical Response System and return to provide care.

When the lone rescuer does not witness the infant casualty going into arrest they should provide two minutes of CPR prior to activating the Emergency Medical Response System.

When activating the Emergency Medical Response System, the rescuer may consider carrying the infant If Injuries permit, and if the distance they must go does not impact on the start or resumption of CPR.

Artificial respiration

The vital organs of the body such as the brain and heart need a continuous supply of oxygen to stay alive. Artificial respiration (AR) is a way you can supply air to the lungs of a casualty who is breathing ineffectively or not breathing at all.

As you breathe, the air you exhale contains enough oxygen to keep a non-breathing person alive. Artificial respiration involves blowing this air into the casualty's lungs to deliver oxygen to the non-breathing person. The number of times you ventilate in one minute is called the rate—AR has to be given at the proper rate to make sure the casualty is getting enough oxygen.

Infants and children with a pulse rate of less than 60 beats per minute and who show signs of poor perfusion despite oxygen and ventilation should receive chest compressions in addition to ventilations.

The methods for ventilating are as follows:

◆ mouth-to-mask with supplemental oxygen

◆ two person bag-valve mask

◆ one person bag-valve mask

Artificial respiration can be given in a wide range of situations. In an emergency situation, keep the following in mind:

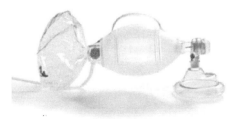

◆ you can start AR right away in any position (but it is best if the casualty is on his back on a firm, flat surface)

◆ you can continue AR while the casualty is being moved to safety by other rescuers

◆ you can give AR for a long time without getting too tired

◆ AR techniques can be used to help a casualty with severe breathing difficulties

Giving AR in some situations, may be more difficult than in others. When this happens, you have to do the best you can (based on your level of training) without putting yourself into danger. Sample situations are:

◆ when severe deforming injuries to the mouth and nose prevent a good seal around the mouth

◆ if blood and/or other body fluids drain into the throat and block the airway, do your best to drain the mouth prior to beginning AR

8

◆ the casualty was poisoned by a toxic gas like hydrogen sulphide and coming in contact with the casualty may result in you being poisoned

◆ the casualty has a corrosive poison on the face or in the mouth, and you don't have a face mask

Health care providers provide artificial respirations to all casualties that have a pulse but are not breathing. Pulse/ breathing checks should be performed every two minutes for at least 5 seconds but no longer than 10 seconds.

With the infant casualty, the rescuer should place a blanket or towel under the torso to prevent the head from being in a hyperflexion position. The infant's head is large and when they are lying on their back on a firm flat surface, unless something is under the upper torso (not including the head) the chin may be forced forward and thus close off the airway.

Bag-valve mask

The bag-valve mask consists of a self-inflating bag, one way valve, face mask and oxygen reservoir. The bag must be connected to oxygen to perform most effectively. With a volume of approximately 1600 mls, the BVM provides less volume than mouth-to-mask.

Two HCPs using the device will be more effective, as HCPs working alone may have difficulty maintaining an airtight seal.

8

General principles for using the bag-valve mask

◆ Position yourself at the top of the casualty's head

◆ Adjunct airways (oral or nasal) may be necessary in conjunction with bag-valve mask if the casualty is unresponsive

◆ After opening and securing the airway, select correct mask size (adult, infant, or child)

◆ Position thumbs over top half of mask, index and middle fingers over the bottom half

◆ Place apex of mask over bridge of nose, then lower mask over mouth and chin. If mask has a large round cuff surrounding a ventilation port, center port over mouth

◆ Use ring and little fingers to bring jaw up to mask

◆ Have an assistant squeeze bag with two hands until chest rises

◆ If alone, form a "C" around the ventilation port with thumb and index finger. Use middle, ring and little fingers under jaw to maintain chin lift and complete the seal. Squeeze the bag with your free hand

◆ Give one ventilation every 5 to 6 seconds for adults and every 3 to 5 seconds for children and infants

◆ If chest does not rise and fall, re-evaluate.

◆ Reposition the head if the chest does not rise.

   ❖ reposition fingers and mask to get a good seal

   ❖ check for obstruction

   ❖ use alternative method (pocket mask) if chest still does not rise

When using the BVM on an infant casualty, be careful not to cover the eyes or chin with the mask.

8

Using advanced airways with masks

When using a pocket or bag valve mask, using an advanced airway is recommended. This involves advanced skill training. If an advanced airway is not available or you are not trained on how to use it, this does not preclude you from using a pocket mask or BVM. Using one or the other without an airway is acceptable. The health care professional may be asked to assist with the bag valve mask when an advanced responder has inserted an advanced airway.

Opening the airway

Health care providers will open a casualty's airway using the head-tilt chin-lift described in Chapter 2. The health care provider has advanced training that includes an alternate method for opening the airway. The jaw thrust without head tilt allows the health care provider to open the airway without moving the head and neck. This method should be used where the rescuer suspects a head or neck injury

Opening and maintaining an airway is a priority. Use the head-tilt chin-lift method if the jaw thrust does not open the airway.

 Using a jaw thrust

1 Place your hands on either side of the head so the head and neck cannot move.

2 Steady your hands on the cheek bones. Grasp the angle of the jaw and lift to open the airway.

3 Open the airway—press on the chin to open the mouth and lift the jaw.

4 Check for signs of breathing and pulse for at least 5 and up to 10 seconds while holding the airway open with the jaw thrust.

5 If there is a pulse, but no breathing, position the mask over the casualty's face. Blow into the casualty's mouth and watch for the chest to rise. Keep lifting the jaw to hold the airway open.

If there is no pulse, begin compressions and continue CPR until an AED arrives on scene.

8

ADULT AND CHILD AR
One rescuer—BVM

1 Position yourself above the casualty's head. Place the mask on the face.

2 Use the thumb and first finger of one hand around valve in a "C" position to press the mask against the face.

3 Use your remaining three fingers in an "E" position to lift up on the jaw.

4 Tilt the head back to open the airway. If the casualty has a suspected head/spinal injury, use a jaw thrust.

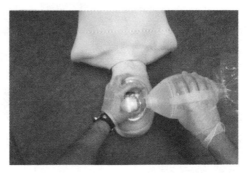

5 Squeeze the bag with your free hand to ventilate. Give each breath in 1 second. Make the chest visibly rise.

◆ adult rescue breathing: 1 breath every 5-6 seconds

◆ child rescue breathing: 1 breath every 3-5 seconds.

6 Check the pulse approximately every 2 minutes.

8

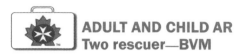

ADULT AND CHILD AR
Two rescuer—BVM

1   Position yourself above the casualty's head. Place the mask on the face.

2   Use the thumb and first finger of EACH hand around the valve in a "C" position. Press the mask against the face.

3   Use the remaining fingers of EACH hand in an "E" position to lift up on the jaw.

4   Tilt the head back to open the airway. If the casualty has a suspected head/spinal injury, use a jaw thrust.

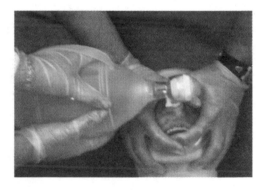

5   Squeeze the bag to ventilate. Give each breath in 1 second. Make the chest visibly rise.

◆ adult rescue breathing: 1 breath every 5-6 sec.

◆ child rescue breathing: 1 breath every 3-5 sec.

6   Check the pulse approximately every 2 minutes.

INFANT AR
One rescuer—BVM

1 Position yourself above the casualty's head.

2 Place a mask over the nose and mouth. Do not cover the eyes or chin.

3 Use the thumb and first finger of one hand around valve in a "C" position to press the mask against the face.

4 Use your remaining three fingers in an "E" position to lift up on the jaw

5 Tilt the head back to open the airway. If the casualty has a suspected head/spinal injury, use a jaw thrust.

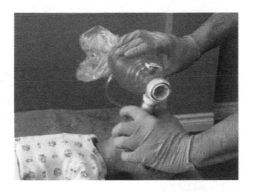

6 Squeeze the bag with your free hand to ventilate.

7 Give each breath in 1 second. Make the chest visibly rise.

8 Give 1 breath every 3-5 seconds (12-20 per minute).

9 Check the pulse approximately every 2 minutes.

INFANT AR
Two rescuer—BVM

1 Position yourself above the casualty's head. Place the mask over the nose and mouth. Do not cover the eyes or chin.

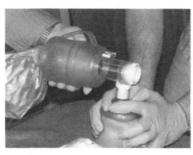

2 Use the thumb and first finger of one hand around the valve in a "C" position. Press the mask against the face.

3 Use the remaining fingers in an "E" position lift up on the jaw.

4 Tilt the head back to open the airway. If the casualty has a suspected head/spinal injury, use a jaw thrust.

5 Squeeze the bag to ventilate. Give each breath in 1 second. Make the chest visibly rise.

6 Give 1 breath every 3-5 seconds (12-20 per minute).

7 Check the pulse approximately every 2 minutes.

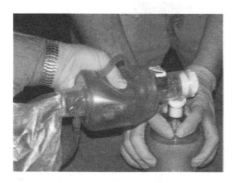

8

How to give assisted breathing

Assisted breathing helps a casualty with severe breathing difficulties to breathe more effectively. It is most useful when the casualty shows very little or no breathing effort. If breathing effort is good, the casualty will likely breathe better on his own. Start assisted breathing when you recognize the signs of severe breathing difficulties.

The technique for assisted breathing is the same as for artificial respiration except for the timing of the ventilations. You seal your mouth around the casualty's mouth and/or nose and blow air into the lungs (use a face mask or shield if you have one). If the casualty is breathing too slowly, give a breath each time the casualty inhales, plus an extra breath in between the casualty's own breaths. Give one breath every five seconds for a total of 12 to 15 breaths per minute.

If the casualty is breathing too fast, give one breath on every second inhalation by the casualty. This will hopefully slow down the casualty's own breathing. Give a total of 12 to 15 breaths per minute.

If the casualty is conscious, explain what you are going to do and why. Reassure the casualty often and encourage him to try to breathe at a good rate with good depth. If the casualty doesn't want you to assist his breathing, explain why it is important. If the casualty still doesn't want you to assist his breathing, don't.

How to give mouth to nose AR

8

Mouth-to-nose AR

Use this method when:

◆ the mouth cannot be opened

◆ there are injuries in or around the mouth, including burns or poisoning

◆ your mouth doesn't fully cover the casualty's mouth, and you can't get a good seal

Mouth-to-nose AR is exactly the same as mouth-to-mouth AR except you hold the mouth closed and you blow into the nose, as shown in the illustration.

Open the casualty's mouth between breaths to help let the air out of the lungs.

Hold the mouth closed.

Blow into the nose—here, a face shield is being used to reduce the risk of infection.

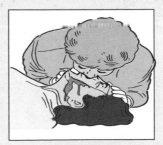

How to give AR to someone who breathes through the neck

Some people breathe through an opening at the base of the neck. This opening, called a stoma, is the result of a previous medical operation called a laryngectomy (lar-en-jec-toe-me).

How to recognize that a person breathes through the neck

You may not know a person breathes through the neck when you try to give AR. If the air seems to go down the airway when you blow, but the chest doesn't rise, check the neck for a stoma. You may also hear air coming out of the stoma as you blow.

Giving AR to a neck breather

The first aid rescue sequence does not change. Once you recognize a person breathes through a stoma, do the following:

◆ expose the entire neck and remove all coverings over the stoma. If there is a tube coming out of the stoma, don't remove it

◆ put a pad under the shoulders to keep them slightly elevated (if you have one close by)

◆ keep the head in line with the body and keep the chin raised

◆ seal the mouth and nose with the hand closest to the head

◆ seal your mouth around the stoma and blow directly into it, or seal your pocket mask over the stoma and blow into the pocket mask

◆ watch the chest rise (look, listen and feel for air movement)

◆ let the air escape from the stoma between breaths

◆ maintain a clean air passage, using a cloth to clean the opening; never use paper tissues

8

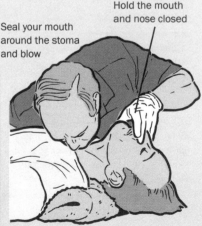

Hold the mouth and nose closed

Seal your mouth around the stoma and blow

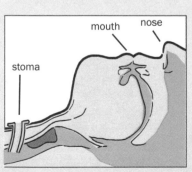

mouth   nose

stoma

Don't blow too hard – gastric distention and vomiting

Gastric distention

If you blow into a casualty at a faster rate than what is recommended or too hard, air will go into the stomach causing the stomach to swell. This is called gastric distention, and it can make it harder to give AR and increase the chances that the casualty will vomit.

If the stomach becomes a little distended, try to prevent further distention by:

◆ repositioning the head and opening the airway again

◆ blowing more slowly, with less air

◆ making sure the airway is held fully open

It is unusual, but the stomach can become so distended that the lungs cannot expand. In this case, the air you blow won't go into the lungs, so you have to relieve the gastric distention by forcing the air in the stomach out. Only relieve gastric distention when the lungs cannot expand and AR is ineffective.

Turn the casualty onto her side with face downwards. Press on her stomach—this should force the air out. The casualty will probably vomit when you do this. If she vomits, quickly wipe out her mouth to keep the airway clear. Reposition the casualty, reassess breathing and pulse, and continue AR if necessary.

To prevent gastric distention

◆ give breaths at the recommended rate

◆ only blow enough air to make the chest rise

◆ make sure the airway is fully open—keep the head tilted well back (but not over-extended)

Vomiting

Vomiting is a common complication both during AR and when the casualty starts to breathe on her own again. If the casualty vomits during AR, turn her to the side and wipe out her mouth. Once the airway is clear, reposition the casualty, reassess breathing and pulse, and continue AR.

If you suspect the casualty has a head or spinal injury, turn her to the side as a unit, so the head and spine stay in the same relative position.

8

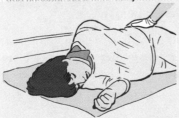
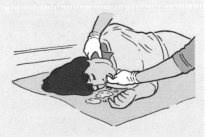

Cardiopulmonary resuscitation (CPR)

Health care providers are expected to have a higher level of knowledge and training. When assessing the casualty, the HCP will check for breathing and a pulse before beginning compressions.

Pulse/Circulation Checks

Health care providers should check for a pulse on all casualties while assessing breathing (see page 52). Rescuers should check the:

Adult—carotid pulse

Child—carotid or femoral pulse

Infant—brachial or femoral pulse

Any child or infant casualty with a pulse rate of less than 60 beats per minute and showing signs of poor perfusion/ circulation, despite oxygen and ventilation, should also receive chest compressions. It is important that the rescuer attempt to use oxygenation and ventilation as the first means of supporting the child or infant. If this is unsuccessful the rescuer will begin compressions. The low heart rate (<60 bpm) does not provide enough circulation to sustain adequate cellular oxygenation; by providing a compression rate of at least 100 compressions per minute the health care provider will assist in providing adequate circulation to an infant or child.

CPR (Compression and Ventilation) Rates

Health care providers will provide the same compression to ventilation rates as the lay rescuer when performing one rescuer CPR for adults, children and infants; as well as two-rescuer adult. The rates will change when they perform two rescuer CPR for the child and infant.

For two rescuer CPR on a child or infant, the rescuer will provide compressions at a rate of 15 compressions to 2 ventilations. Depth of compressions should be at least 1/3 the depth of the infant or child's chest with a rate of at least 100 compressions per minute.

In the case of the infant casualty, the rescuer may encircle the infant casualty's chest and use their thumbs side by side or one on top of the other to provide compressions. The method used will depend on the size of the infant casualty and the rescuer's thumbs.

Advanced Airways

There are a number of advanced airways used by professional rescuers including an endotracheal tube (ETI), laryngeal mask airway (LMA) and combitube.

When an advanced airway is being used during two-rescuer CPR, the rescuers do not have to worry about synchronizing breaths to compressions. This means that the rescuers will not have to worry about pausing between chest compressions for ventilations. When an advanced airway is in place, the rate of ventilation will be one breath every 6 to 8 seconds for all age categories as compressions are given.

8

ADULT CPR/AED

Begin ESM. Check breathing and pulse for at least 5 and no more than 10 seconds. If there is a pulse, but no breathing, begin artificial respiration. If there is no pulse, begin compressions.

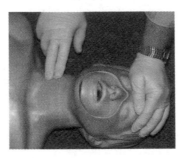

One rescuer 30:2

◆ Give 30 chest compressions in the middle of the upper chest using two hands.

◆ Push hard, push fast (100 x per min) to a depth of at least 2 inches (5 cm). The pressure and release phases take the same time. Release pressure and completely remove your weight at the top of each compression to allow chest to return to the resting position after each compression. Minimize interruptions.

◆ Give 2 breaths.

◆ Continue 30:2 until:

❖ an AED is ready for use

❖ EMS/advanced providers arrive or

❖ the casualty shows signs of recovery.

Two or more rescuers 30:2

◆ Rescuer one—30 chest compressions at a rate of 100 x per minute.

◆ Rescuer two—give 2 rescue breaths, enough to make the chest visibly rise.

◆ Quickly change positions every 5 cycles (2 minutes)

◆ if advanced airway in place—one breath every 6-8 seconds. No pause in compressions for breaths.

Defibrillation

◆ Expose the chest. Turn on the AED. Follow the voice prompts. Select and attach the adult pads.

◆ SHOCK advised—CLEAR and give 1 shock. Immediately resume chest compressions.

◆ NO SHOCK advised—Immediately resume chest compressions.

◆ Continue 30 compressions—2 breaths for 5 cycles (approx. 2 minutes). Analyse heart rhythm, continue CPR/AED until advanced providers take over.

8

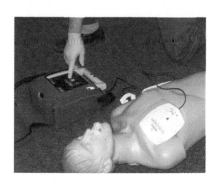

CHILD CPR/AED

Begin ESM. Check breathing and pulse for at least 5 and no more than 10 seconds. If there is a pulse, but no breathing, begin artificial respiration. If there is no pulse or if the pulse rate is less than 60 beats per minute with poor perfusion, begin compressions.

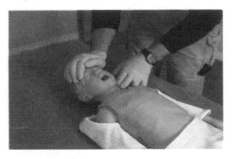

One rescuer 30:2

◆ Give 30 chest compressions in the middle of the upper chest using one or two hands.

◆ Push hard, push fast (at least 100 x per min) to a depth of about 2 inches (5 cm) or 1/3 of the depth of the chest. The pressure and release phases take the same time. Release pressure and completely remove your weight at the top of each compression to allow chest to return to the resting position after each compression. Minimize interruptions

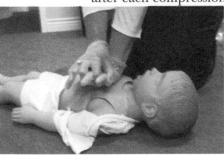

◆ Give 2 breaths.

◆ Continue 30 compressions: 2 breaths. If alone call EMS after 5 cycles (approx. 2 minutes).

8

2 or more rescuers (15:2)

◆ Rescuer one—15 chest compressions at a rate of at least 100 x per minute.

◆ Rescuer two—give 2 rescue breaths, enough to make the chest visibly rise.

◆ Quickly change positions every 10 cycles (2 minutes).

◆ if advanced airway in place: one breath every 6-8 seconds with no pause in compressions

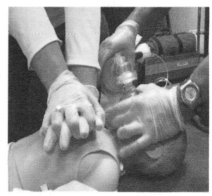

Defibrillation

◆ Expose the chest. Turn on the AED. Follow the voice prompts. Select and attach the pediatric pads. If pediatric pads are not available, use adult pads.

◆ SHOCK advised: CLEAR and give 1 shock. Immediately resume chest compressions.

◆ NO SHOCK advised: Immediately resume chest compressions.

◆ Continue 15 compressions—2 breaths for 5 cycles (approx. 2 minutes). Analyse heart rhythm, continue CPR/AED until advanced providers take over.

8

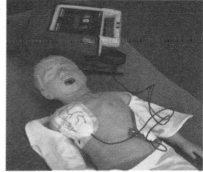

Infant CPR/AED

Begin ESM. Check breathing and pulse for at least 5 and no more than 10 seconds. If there is a pulse, but no breathing, begin artificial respiration. If there is no pulse or if the pulse rate is less than 60 beats per minute with poor perfusion, begin compressions.

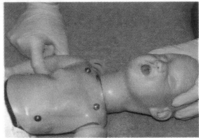

One rescuer (30:2)

◆ Give 30 chest compressions using two fingers, just below the nipple line.

◆ Push hard, push fast (at least 100 x per min) to a depth of about 1 1/2 inches (4 cm) or 1/3 of the depth of the chest. The pressure and release phases take the same time. Release pressure and completely remove your weight at the top of each compression to allow chest to return to the resting position after each compression. Minimize interruptions.

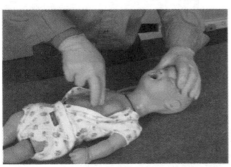

◆ Give 2 breaths.

◆ Continue 30 compressions: 2 breaths. If alone call EMS after 5 cycles (approx. 2 minutes).

2 or more rescuers (15:2)

◆ Rescuer one—15 chest compressions (2 thumbs with the fingers encircling the chest) at a rate of at least 100 x per minute.

◆ Rescuer two—2 rescue breaths, enough to make chest visibly rise.

◆ Quickly change positions every 10 cycles (2 minutes).

◆ if advanced airway in place: one breath every 6-8 seconds with no pause in compressions for breaths.

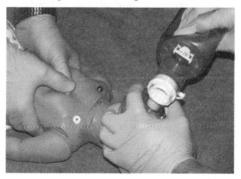

Defibrillation

◆ Expose the chest, turn on the AED. Follow the voice prompts. Select and attach the pediatric pads. If pediatric pads are not available, use adult pads. Be sure the pads to not touch each other.

◆ SHOCK advised: CLEAR and give 1 shock. Immediately resume chest compressions.

◆ NO SHOCK advised: Immediately resume chest compressions.

◆ Continue 15 compressions—2 breaths for 5 cycles (approx. 2 minutes). Analyse heart rhythm, continue CPR/AED until advanced providers take over.

8

Using an AED

The health care provider has a stronger medical background than the lay rescuer and is therefore expected to be able to more accurately and efficiently use the automated external defibrillator in a situation where a casualty is in cardiac arrest and CPR is being provided.

Health care providers should be taught to work in teams. When a two rescuer team is available, one rescuer provides CPR right away and the second rescuer obtains and uses the AED. This is the optimal situation as the rescuers have the ability to provide ongoing CPR prior to defibrillation.

The rescuers should minimize interruptions of CPR for the application of the AED. In the case of an unwitnessed, prolonged response time or asphyxial arrest the should provide two minutes of CPR prior to defibrillation.

The pediatric AED system/pads are to be used only on infants and children (as defined on page 337); when using an AED on older children the rescuer will use adult size pads and energy. Also, if a pediatric AED system is not available the rescuer should use the adult system.

A common theme that will occur for the health care provider is that they will provide two minutes of CPR post "shock" or "no shock" on all casualties unless that casualty shows obvious signs of life or Advanced Life Support arrives to take over care.

If Advanced Life Support arrives to take over care, the health care provider should follow the direction set by the ALS provider. Otherwise the health care provider will use the AED based on the following circumstances:

8

Adult (One Rescuer) Unwitnessed Arrest

In this case attach the AED and use it as soon as possible.

Adult (One Rescuer) Prolonged Response

If the rescuer takes longer than four to five minutes to reach the adult casualty, he may provide two minutes of CPR prior to attaching the AED and using it (follow local protocols).

Adult (One Rescuer) Asphyxial Arrest

In this case, the rescuer should provide two minutes of CPR prior to attaching the AED and using it. CPR is performed for two minutes first to help correct the cause of the arrest.

Adult (One Rescuer) Witnessed Arrest

In this case the rescuer should use the AED immediately without performing any CPR. There is a four to five minute window from the time of witnessed arrest to the time of defibrillation, before CPR must be performed.

8

Adult (Two Rescuer)

When a two rescuer team is available, one rescuer should begin CPR right away and the second rescuer should obtain and use the AED. This is the optimal situation as the rescuers have the ability to provide uninterrupted CPR prior to defibrillation.

The rescuers should minimize interruptions of CPR during the set up and application of the AED. In the case of an unwitnessed, prolonged response time or asphyxial arrest provide two minutes of CPR prior to defibrillation.

If the arrest is witnessed and the AED arrives within four to five minutes, CPR should be started by one rescuer and the AED applied by the second rescuer. As soon as the AED is applied allow the AED to analyze the rhythm.

Child/Infant (One Rescuer) Unwitnessed or Prolonged Arrest

In this case the rescuer may provide two minutes of CPR prior to attaching the AED and using it (follow local protocols).

Child/Infant (One Rescuer) Witnessed Arrest

In this case, the rescuer should use the AED immediately without performing any CPR. There is a four to five minute window from the time of witnessed arrest to the time of defibrillation, before CPR must be performed.

Child/Infant (Two Rescuer)

When a two rescuer team is available, one rescuer should begin to perform CPR right away and the second rescuer should obtain and use the AED. This is the optimal situation as the rescuers have the ability to provide uninterrupted CPR prior to defibrillation.

The rescuers should minimize interruptions of CPR during the set up and application of the AED. In the case of an unwitnessed, prolonged response time or asphyxial arrest, the rescuers should provide two minutes of CPR prior to defibrillation.

If the arrest is witnessed and the AED arrives within four to five minutes, CPR should be started by one rescuer and the AED applied by the second rescuer. As soon as the AED is applied allow the AED to analyze the rhythm.

Team Approach

In most EMS and health care environments, there is increased emphasis on providing CPR and AED as a team effort. When multiple rescuers are available and an AED is at the scene, rescuers should work as a team to provide uninterrupted CPR and AED. While one rescuer assesses the casualty and prepares to start CPR, the second rescuer sets up the AED. If a third rescuer is available, this person sets up the bag-valve mask and prepares to deliver ventilations. One of the most important considerations when integrating CPR and AED is to reduce the intervals between stopping chest compressions and the delivery of a shock as well as the interval between the delivery of the shock and the resumption of chest compressions.

Post Resuscitation

In some cases, the casualty will regain a pulse. This is exciting, however the casualty is still in serious condition. In caring for a casualty whose pulse has returned, remember:

◆ Monitor the pulse carefully, for it may diminish

◆ It is common for casualties to not breathe even though a pulse has returned; ventilate or assist with ventilations as necessary

◆ If the casualty has regained a pulse and has adequate respirations and has not been injured, place him or her in a recovery position

◆ Apply high-concentration oxygen if you are trained and allowed to do so by local protocol

◆ Keep the AED attached to the casualty

◆ Your assessment of the casualty's condition should be ongoing until you hand over care

8

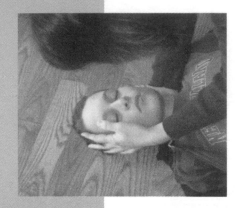

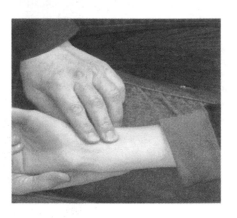

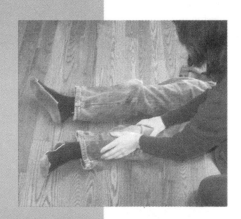

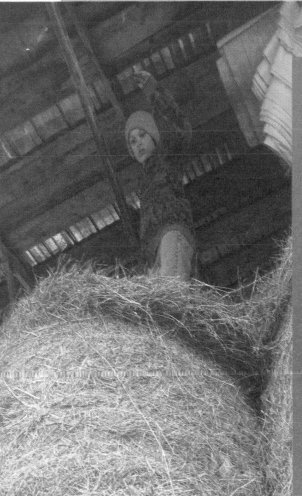

QUICK REFERENCE

Emergency scene management summary

Emergency scene management has many steps and can be quite complicated, but the initial scene survey, primary survey and the start of life-saving first aid usually happens very quickly—within one or two minutes. This summary shows all the steps on four pages and gives an idea of the flow of steps.

Scene survey

Take charge of the situation.

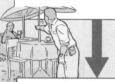

Call out for help to attract bystanders.

Assess hazards and make the area safe.

Find out the history of the scene, how many casualties there are and the mechanism(s) of injury.

Identify yourself as a first aider and offer to help.

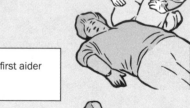

Assess responsiveness

Send, or go for medical help.

Primary survey

Don't move the casualty to do the primary survey unless you absolutely have to. Give first aid for life-threatening conditions as you find them while checking the ABCs.

Responsive casualty

A Check the airway

Ask "What happened?" How well the casualty answers tells you if the airway is clear.

B Check for effective breathing

If breathing is effective. . .

C Check circulation

◆ control obvious, severe bleeding

◆ check for shock by checking skin condition and temperature

◆ check with a rapid body survey for hidden, severe, external bleeding and signs of internal bleeding

Unresponsive casualty

A Open the airway

Use the head-tilt chin-lift (or jaw-thrust without head-tilt if trained). If you suspect a spinal injury, check breathing, before opening the airway.

B Check for breathing

For at least 5 and no more than 10 seoonds

If breathing appears ineffective. . .or absent

C Circulation

◆ begin CPR with 30 compressions

◆ open the airway

◆ give two breaths and continue cycles of 30 compressions and two breaths

◆ apply a defibrillator as soon as available

A

Secondary survey

After giving first aid for life-threatening injuries, do a secondary survey if medical help is delayed, you have to transport the casualty or the casualty has more than one injury.

1. History of the casualty

S   symptoms
A   allergies
M   medications
P   past and present medical history
L   last meal
E   events leading to the incident

2. Assess the vital signs

level of consciousness
breathing
pulse
skin temperature

3. Head-to-toe examination

check the head   check the neck   check both collarbones

check the shoulders, arms and hands   check the chest and under   check the abdomen and under

check the pelvis and buttocks   check the legs, ankles and feet

4. Give first aid. . .

. . . for injuries or illnesses found

Ongoing Casualty Care

Instruct a bystander to maintain manual support of the head and neck, if head/spinal injuries are suspected.

Continue to steady and support any injuries manually, if needed.

Give first aid for shock
- reassure the casualty
- loosen tight clothing
- place the casualty in the best position for the condition
- cover the casualty to preserve body heat

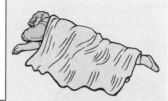

Monitor the casualty's condition
- check the ABCs often
- give nothing by mouth

Record the events of the situation
- protect the casualty's belongings

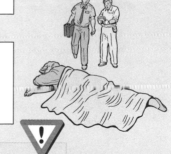

Report on what happened
- tell whoever takes over what happened and what first aid has been given

A

Do not leave the casualty until you hand control of the scene over to someone else.

Assessing level of consciousness

A first aider uses the Modified Glasgow Coma Scale to assess and describe levels of consciousness. The scale is based on the casualty's ability:

◆ to open the eyes—this is the eye opening response

◆ to speak—this is the verbal response

◆ to move muscles—this is the motor response

Use the information below to determine whether the casualty is conscious, semi-conscious or unconscious.

	When a person is conscious. . .	When a person is semi-conscious. . .	When the person is unconscious. . .
Eye opening response	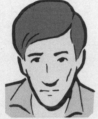 . . . eyes open spontaneously	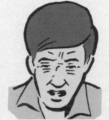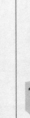 . . . eyes open to speech or pain	. . . eyes don't open
Verbal response	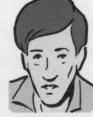 . . . he is oriented and alert	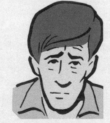 . . . he is confused, doesn't make sense	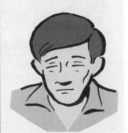 . . . he is not aware of his surroundings
Motor response	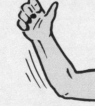 . . . he obeys commands	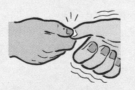 . . . he reacts to pain but does not obey comands	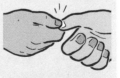 . . . he doesn't react to pain

A

Sample first aid report form

First Aid Report

First aider   Date _____

Location _____

Name _____

Address _____

City _____

Province _____ Postal code _____

Telephone number _____

Casualty

Name _____

Address _____

City _____

Province _____ Postal code _____

Telephone number _____

☐ Male   ☐ Female   Age (approx.) _____

Scene survey

Type of incident _____

Number of casualties _____
(use a separate form for each casualty)

Casualty responsiveness
    ☐ responsive   ☐ unresponsive

Primary survey

Airway
    ☐ clear
    ☐ partly blocked
    ☐ completely blocked

Breathing
    ☐ yes... ☐ effective   ☐ ineffective
    ☐ no

Circulation
    Pulse   ☐ yes   ☐ no
    Severe bleeding ☐ yes   ☐ no
    Shock   ☐ yes   ☐ no

Secondary survey

History
    Symptoms _____
    _____
    Allergies _____
    Medications _____
    Past medical history _____
    Last meal _____
    Events leading to incident _____
    _____

Vital signs
    Time taken   ____   ____   ____
    Level of consc.   ____   ____   ____
    Breathing rate   ____   ____   ____
    Breathing rhythm ____   ____   ____
    Breathing depth   ____   ____   ____
    Pulse rate   ____   ____   ____
    Pulse rhythm   ____   ____   ____
    Pulse strength   ____   ____   ____
    Skin cond./temp. ____   ____   ____

Head-to-toe examination
    Head _____
    Neck _____
    Collarbones _____
    Shoulders arms/hands _____
    Chest and under _____
    Abdomen and under _____
    Pelvis and buttocks _____
    Legs/feet _____

First aid given

_____
_____
_____
_____

Hand over to medical help

_____
_____
_____

A

Quick first aid reference

Send for an ambulance as soon as there is indication of a life-threatening emergency:

◆ loss of consciousness

◆ breathing difficulty or stopped breathing

◆ impaired circulation (severe bleeding, signs of cardiac emergency)

Signs and symptoms   First aid

Allergic reaction

Itchy, flushed skin	Position casualty at rest
Sneezing, runny nose	If casualty has medication, help her to take it
Swelling of the airway	Monitor consciousness and breathing
Nausea, vomiting	Get medical help

Angina

Denial, sense of impending doom	Position casualty at rest
Heaviness, tightness in chest	If casualty has medication, help her to take it
Indigestion, aching jaw	Monitor consciousness and breathing
Pale skin, sweating	Get medical help

Asthma

Shortness of breath with coughing or wheezing	Position casualty for comfort sitting or semi-sitting
Sitting upright, trying to breathe	Assist with medication
Blue colour to face (cyanosis)	Monitor consciousness and breathing
Anxiety, tightness in chest	Get medical help

Bites and stings

Pain at site	Position casualty at rest
Heat and swelling at site	Remove stinger if appropriate
Redness, itching	Clean affected area
Rash or bumps on skin	Monitor consciousness and breathing

Bleeding (external)

Obvious wound	Apply pressure
External blood	Position casualty at rest
Cold, clammy skin	When bleeding stops, clean the area
Restlessness, apprehension	Apply dressings and bandages
Faintness, dizziness	Check circulation

Bleeding (internal)

No obvious wound	Shock position
Blood from ears, nose, in urine/stool	If thirsty, moisten lips
Bloodshot or black eye(s)	Monitor consciousness and breathing
Blood coughed up or in vomitus	Get medical help

Burns

Skin red to pearly white or charred	Position casualty at rest
Pain in mild cases, no pain if severe	Cool the affected area
Blisters	Apply dressings and bandages
Moist skin, dry leathery if severe	Check circulation

Choking

Mild obstruction — Stay with casualty

Able to speak	Encourage casualty to cough
Signs of distress	If obstruction not cleared, get medical help
Red face	

Severe obstruction — Position yourself supporting the casualty

Not able to speak	Give 5 back blows, 5 abdominal thrusts
Weak or no coughing	Check mouth
Grey face, blue lips, ears	Be prepared for loss of consciousness

A

Concussion

Partial or complete loss of consciousness usually of short duration	If you suspect head/spinal injury, do not move casualty
Shallow breathing, nausea	Monitor consciousness and breathing
Pale, sweating, headache	Get medical help

Diabetic Emergency

Hypoglycemia (needs sugar) — Position casualty at rest

Sweaty, pale, cold — Give sugar

Headache, trembling — Monitor consciousness and breathing

Confusion, irritable, aggressive — If no improvement, get medical help

Hyperglycemia (needs insulin) — Position casualty at rest

Flushed, dry, warm — If unsure, whether hyper or hypo, give sugar

Drowsy, becoming unconscious — Monitor consciousness and breathing

Thirsty, breath smells like nail polish — If no improvement, get medical help

Embedded object

Obvious wound — Position casualty at rest

Object visible in wound — Build up dressings around object

(Do not remove embedded object) — Apply dressings without pressure on object

Bleeding at wound site — Bandage get medical help

Emergency Childbirth

Longer and stronger contractions — Position casualty at rest

Mother tells you the baby is coming — Keep casualty warm

Straining, bearing down — Place sanitary napkin or clean pad for bleeding

Feeling she has to have bowel movement — Get medical help

A

Fainting

Pale, sweaty — Position casualty at rest

Dizzy and nauseous — Loosen tight clothing, get fresh air

Unsteady, may collapse — Stay with casualty until fully recovered

Frostbite

White waxy skin — Get casualty out of cold

Skin firm but soft underneath — Position casualty

Skin becomes cold and hard — Rewarm affected area

Painful at first, then numb — Give first aid for wounds

Head/spinal injury

Confused, lightheaded	Tell casualty not to move
Mechanism of injury to suggest	Monitor responsiveness and breathing
Pale, cold, clammy	Get medical help

Heart attack

(see Angina)

	If conscious, position casualty at rest
Denial, sense of impending doom	Position casualty at rest
Heaviness, tightness in chest	If casualty has medication, help her to take it
Indigestion, aching jaw	Monitor consciousness and breathing
Pale skin, sweating	Get medical help
Unconsciousness	**If unresponsive** and not breathing,
Stopped breathing	Get medical help, and send for AED
	Begin CPR

Hypothermia

Shivering gets worse, then stops	Get casualty out of cold
Breathing slows, and may stop	Position casualty at rest
Confused, sleepy, irrational may lose consciousness	Rewarm casualty

Heat exhaustion

Excessive sweating, dilated pupils	Get casualty out of heat
Dizziness, blurred vision, headache, cramps	Give as much to drink as she will take
Cold, clammy skin, shallow breathing	Remove excessive clothing
Possible loss of consciousness	Monitor responsiveness and breathing

A

Heatstroke

Body temperature hot to touch	Get casualty out of heat
Skin flushed, hot and may be wet or dry	Remove excess clothing
Restless, headache, dizziness	Immersion in cold water
Vomiting, convulsions, unconsciousness	Stay with the casualty, get medical help

Poisoning

Swallowed

nausea, vomiting,

discolouration at lips, burns

Absorbed

Red skin, blisters, swelling, burns

Injected

Irritation at point of entry

Inhaled

Trouble breathing, chest pain

Position casualty

Conscious casualty - call Poison Control

Unconscious casualty - get medical help

If powder, brush off

Flush area with large amounts of water

Monitor consciousness and breathing

Get medical help

Ensure safety of yourself and others

Get casualty away from hazard, give first aid

Seizure

Sudden cry

Stiffening of body

Loss of consciousness, causing
casualty to fall

Body jerks

Breathing irregular or stopped

Loss of bladder or bowel control

Do not interfere during seizure

Protect casualty from injury

When seizure in complete,
position conscious casualty at rest

unconscious casualty in recovery position

Monitor consciousness and breathing

Get medical help

Stroke

F.A.S.T.

Complains of sudden weakness

Symptoms related to affected area

Dizziness, headache

Position conscious casualty at rest

Give nothing by mouth

Monitor consciousness and breathing

Get medical help

Unconsciousness

Eyes do not open

Does not respond to instructions

Does not respond to touch

**Indicates worsening of existing
condition**

Get medical help

Give first aid for injuries or illness

Position casualty in recovery position

Monitor breathing and begin CPR if needed

A

Cardiopulmonary Resuscitation

Assess responsivenss

If unresponsive, send someone to call for medical help and get an AED. Check breathing for at least 5 and not more than 10 seconds. If not breathing:

Begin compressions

Adult	Child	Infant
	Position directly over centre of the chest	
Use two hands	Use one or two hands	Use two fingers
Compress 2 inches (5 cm)	Compress 1/3 depth of the casualty's chest	

PUSH HARD   PUSH FAST

Compression at a rate of at
least 100 per minute

Give 30 compressions

Open airway and give two breaths

Continue CPR at ratio of 30 compressions to 2 breaths until:

medical help arrives

someone else takes over, or

you are to exhausted to continue

Apply AED as soon as it is available

Turn on AED and follow machine

A

Additional rescue carries

The most common carries are presented in Chapter 2 in the section on Lifting and Carrying. In some cases, these carries may not be appropriate. Additional carries are presented here. Always be aware of the risk to both the first aider and the casualty, and the increased danger if a casualty suddenly loses consciousness.

Pick-a-back

This carry is used for a conscious casualty with lower limb injuries, provided he can use his arms. The casualty must be able to help get into position on your back or be already seated at chair or table height.

1 Crouch with your back between the casualty's knees.

2 Have the casualty hold on around your neck.

3 Support the casualty's legs and lift. Use your leg muscles to stand up, keeping your back straight.

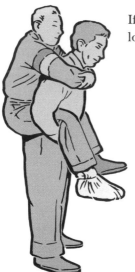

If the casualty is to be carried pick-a-back for a long distance, make a carrying seat.

◆ Make a large adjustable loop from a strap or belts. Put your arms through the loop, arranging it behind your neck and down the front of your shoulders. Leave the bottom half of the loop free at the back about the level of your buttocks

◆ Pass the casualty's legs through the bottom of the loop; one on each side. Position the loop under the casualty's buttocks, adjusting it for a good carrying position and proper weight distribution

Cradle carry

Use the cradle carry to lift children and lightweight adults.

1 Kneel on one knee at the casualty's side.

2 Place the casualty's arm around your neck as you support the back and shoulders.

3 Pass your other arm under the knees to grasp the thighs.

4 Ensure a solid footing and place the feet apart for good balance.

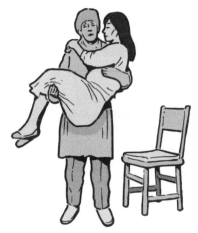

A

5 Lift using your legs, keep your back straight, and your abdominal muscles tense.

Fire fighter's carry

The fire fighter's carry is used for casualties who are helpless and are not too heavy for the rescuer.

1   With the casualty lying face up in front of you, stand with your toes against the casualty's toes. Grasp her wrists and pull her upward and forward.

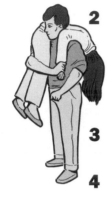

2   Maintain a grip on one wrist as you turn and bend to catch the casualty's upper body across your shoulder. The lifting manoeuvre is a continuous, smooth motion to bring the casualty through a sitting position to an upright position, finishing with the casualty draped over your shoulder.

3   Adjust the weight across your shoulders, with the casualty's legs straddling your shoulder.

4   Pass your arm between the casualty's legs and grasp her wrist. This will stabilize the casualty on your shoulders and leave your other hand free.

Two-hand seat

A casualty, who is unable to support his upper body, can be carried by two rescuers, using the two-hand seat.

1   The rescuers crouch on either side of the casualty.

2   Each rescuer reaches across the casualty's back to grasp his clothing at the waist on the opposite side.

3   Each rescuer passes his other hand under the thighs, keeping his fingers bent and holding padding to protect against the fingernails. Hook the bent fingers together to form a rigid seat. Alternatively, the rescuers can hold each other's wrists.

4   The rescuers lift with their legs, keeping their backs straight. Once in the standing position, the rescuers adjust their hands and arms for comfort. When the casualty is securely positioned, the bearers step off together, each using the inside foot.

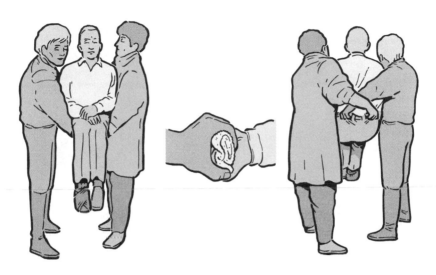

Four-hand seat

A conscious casualty who can use his hands and arms can be carried on a four-hand seat by two rescuers.

A

1   Each rescuer grasps his own left wrist with his right hand, then grasps the right wrist of the other rescuer with his left hand to form a square.

2   Tell the casualty to put his arms around the rescuers' shoulders and hoist himself up to permit the bearers to pass their hands under the buttocks to position them under the thighs at a point of balance.

3   Instruct the casualty to hold onto the rescuers' shoulders to keep his balance and support his upper body.

4   The bearers step off together, each using the inside
foot.

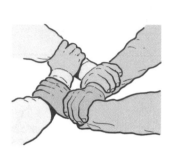

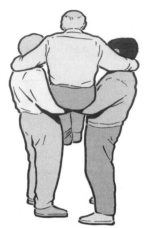

Using a blanket with a stretcher

A casualty can be wrapped on a stretcher so that a blanket
provides maximum warmth with minimum weight on the
casualty. It will also allow easy access to the casualty's wounds
if that is necessary during transportation.

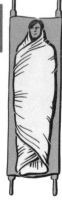

1   Place a blanket on the stretcher under the casualty
with diagonally opposite corners at the head and
feet.

2   Place padding at appropriate places on the blanket
to fill the natural hollows at the casualty's neck and
back. Centre the casualty on the blanket.

3   Cover the feet with the bottom corner and bring
the corner at the head around the neck to the
chest. Wrap the legs and lower body with one
side. Tuck in the last corner on the opposite side.

Using a short spine board

A short spine board is used to immobilize the head, neck and upper spine while the casualty is in a sitting position. They are especially useful for removing a casualty with a suspected head and/or spinal injury from a motor vehicle following a crash.

Two rescuers are needed to use a short spine board. The first rescuer, who can be a bystander, supports the casualty, holding the head and neck in a rigid position as shown by the first aider. The second rescuer, the first aider, completes the immobilization onto the short spine board.

◆ Position the short spine board along the back of the casualty with the bottom edge below the pelvis and the headpiece at least level with the top of the head. All natural hollows of the body must be padded. Pad both sides of the head to prevent rotation.

◆ Secure the casualty's head to the board and the casualty's arms to the sides. Secure the chest and lower trunk to the board.

Commercial spine boards and extrication devices are available. If you have access to these materials, be sure you are properly trained in their use. Always follow the manufacturer's instructions.

A short spine board is better than no spine board, but to fully immobilize the head and neck, use a hard cervical collar (see page 283).

When the casualty is removed from a sitting position on a short spine board, immobilize him and the short spine board onto a long spine board, then transport.

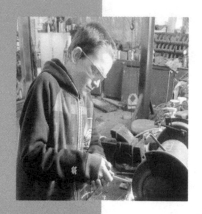

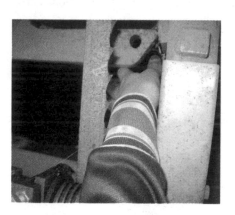

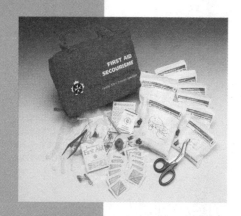

B

BE SAFE, BE PREPARED

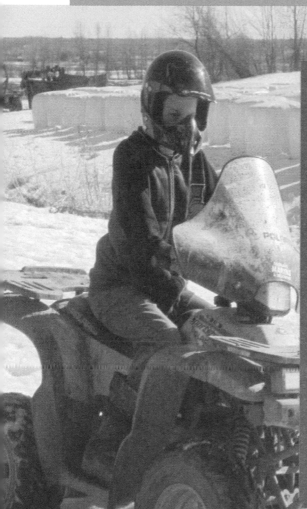

- ◆ *Safety tips about coming home alone*

- ◆ *Familiarize members of family with safety routes in case of fire*

- ◆ *Tips on childproofing your home*

- ◆ *Safety tips for seniors*

- ◆ *Workplace safety*

- ◆ *Road safety*

- ◆ *Be prepared!*

You can't make all things safe all of the time, but you can make most things safe most of the time. And when things aren't safe, you can recognize them and avoid the hazards. It's usually more than one factor that contributes to an injury. For instance, consider the combination of an unsafe situation, a tired person and poor lighting conditions. Individually, the chance of injury is low. But together, it's almost a sure thing.

Learn to recognize combinations of factors that can lead to injury—this is your safety sense. It goes beyond simply doing this and that in the name of safety—it means thinking on your feet all of the time, recognizing potential injury situations and doing something about them. Taking a first aid course will help to develop your safety sense. Research has shown that people with first aid training have fewer injuries. Make safety a habit. Once you've got it, it'll rub off on those around you.

Personal safety

Safety when leaving home

Make a plan of where you are going. Tell someone your plan, where you can be reached and when you expect to return. Tell her what to do, and when, if you don't return by your expected time.

Safety when coming home

If you are coming home and suspect you are being followed:

◆ do not go into your house if no one is home

◆ go to a busy area, like a shopping mall or restaurant, where there are other people to help you if needed. If you are not near a public place, go to a home where lights are on and it looks as if someone is home. Telephone someone you know. Explain the situation and have them meet you

◆ call the police immediately if you continue to be concerned

Don't take risks regarding your personal safety. If you are in an unfamiliar neighbourhood or city, play it safe.

B

Safety at home

If safety isn't a regular topic of conversation in your home, now is a great time to make it one. Talk about how to deal with possible emergencies. This prepares everyone. Talk with children about how to recognize an emergency and what to do. Talk about the people in your community who are trustworthy and can help, including block parents, store clerks and teachers.

Replace old smoke detectors with new ones every 10 years.

Fire safety

Many, many homes and lives are lost to fires each year. Take the time today to look for, and eliminate, fire hazards in your home. Start with the following:

◆ do you have rules about smoking in your house?

◆ do you have smoke detectors between the living areas and sleeping areas of your home. Do you test them once a month and change the batteries once a year?

◆ is the electrical wiring in good repair?

◆ are matches and lighters kept in a safe place, out of reach of children?

◆ are flammable materials safely stored?

Prepare—even with the finest prevention program, your family must always be ready for a fire. Everyone should know what to do in case of a fire. This includes knowing where fire extinguishers are and how to use them.

Visit your local fire station

Your local fire station can provide you with all you need to take action to prevent fires in your home. They are in the business of fire prevention and are happy to help you.

B

Plan—make an escape plan of what to do if there is a fire. Include a meeting place where everyone is to go if there is a fire, such as a tree in the neighbour's yard.

Protect—in case of fire do the following:

◆ remain calm and stop whatever you are doing

◆ use your escape plan to get out quickly and safely— close doors and windows behind you to help stop the fire from spreading

9-1-1

9-1-1 is the emergency phone number in many communities

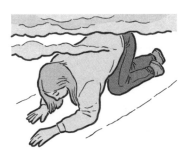

Keep your head low and crawl under the smoke

◆ go immediately to your meeting place

◆ send one person to call for help

◆ don't go back inside for anything— possessions aren't worth the cost of a life and many lives have been lost this way

B

Safety for young children

Here (at home)

The easiest and most effective way to make your home safe for young children is to get down on your hands and knees and have a good look around from your child's perspective. Use your child's point of view—be curious and search for new and exciting adventures. Especially beware of everyday items that could be fatal to a child (window blind cords, electrical cords, appliances and poisonous houseplants).

There (when you aren't there to help)

Teach youngsters skills that are important in an emergency. As early as possible teach your children:

◆ their address and telephone number

◆ your proper names ("mommy" and "daddy" don't help in an emergency)

◆ how to use the local emergency phone numbers— make sure they know how to use them properly

◆ how to use a pay telephone—remember that you don't need money to call emergency services

What is an emergency?

Talk to your children about emergencies and discuss specific examples. Explain that there are many different types of emergencies. Talk about what to do if:

◆ they lose a favourite toy

◆ the cat gets stuck in a neighbour's tree

◆ a friend falls and cuts his knee

◆ mommy or daddy falls down and can't get up

◆ they see a fire in the house

Teach your children basic safety rules. Very young children can learn to recognize dangerous situations. They can also understand what they should do in an emergency. As children grow, give them more and more responsibility. Get them involved in your regular safety check-ups.

B

Safety for seniors

Falls

Falls are a common cause of injury for seniors, often resulting in serious emergencies. This is partly because bones become more fragile as we get older. Relatively minor injuries can become serious and perhaps life threatening. Take action to prevent falls (see below).

Medications

Medications present many potential hazards. Dispose of unused prescriptions and expired over-the-counter medications. Contact your local pharmacy as they may take care of them for you. Remember the following tips when taking medications:

◆ do not take prescription medication intended for someone else

◆ always keep medications in their original containers with the dosage and the instructions clearly indicated

◆ write down when prescription medicines are taken, so you can refer back, if required, at a later time

B

Preventing falls

◆ secure all rugs and carpets
◆ use secure foot stools to reach high places (cupboards, shelves)
◆ use non-slip mats in the bathtub or shower
◆ use handrails when climbing and descending stairs
◆ don't take risks—don't use a stool when you know you should use a ladder; don't carry too many parcels at a time—better safe than sorry!

◆ if you have any questions about your medication, call your doctor or pharmacist right away—they're there to help

Safety when living alone

Seniors often live alone. If you live alone, make sure you have a plan in place in case something happens. If you fell and were injured this evening, how long would it be before someone came to look for you?

If you have a routine activity such as work or school, someone may notice your absence. But if you don't have a regular routine, arrange to speak to a certain person every day. The contact can be with anyone, and it can be short and simple. Two people, each living alone, can check in on each other. If one does not hear from the other at the right time, she gets help right away.

B

Safety at work

Safety in the workplace is the responsibility of everyone involved. Take time to assess your situation. Recognize that the specific hazards, and what you can do about them, depend on the nature of your work.

Management should. . .

◆ meet and exceed the occupational health and safety regulations for all aspects of the workplace

◆ actively promote a safe attitude

◆ establish procedures to encourage employees to report safety concerns

◆ have, and practise, an emergency evacuation plan

Employees should. . .

◆ know the occupational health and safety regulations that affect your jobs

◆ collaborate with employers in improving workplace safety

◆ encourage safety among the people you work with, and discourage unsafe acts

◆ use the personal protective equipment provided to you

◆ report unsafe conditions

◆ learn about, and use, safe and healthy work practices, including: following safety rules, using

B

Make the place safe

Develop a workplace floor plan including location of:

◆ emergency exits
◆ sprinkler systems
◆ hazardous materials/ chemicals
◆ valuable equipment (computer systems etc)
◆ information on key personnel to contact in case of emergency

proper procedures for lifting heavy items, working at ergonomic workstations and using equipment designed to help with potentially dangerous activities, like using a cart or dolly to move a heavy item.

WHMIS

The Workplace Hazardous Materials Information System (WHMIS) is used to identify hazardous materials and to help workers protect themselves from real dangers. WHMIS includes labelling products with supplier labels and workplace labels, and having a material safety data sheet (MSDS) available for each hazardous product in the workplace.

Supplier label—these are put on by the supplier of the product. They include:

◆ product identifier

◆ risk phrases

◆ precautionary measures

◆ first aid measures

◆ supplier identifiers

◆ class symbol(s)

◆ reference to MSDS being available

◆ English and French information

◆ a distinct hatchmark border in a contrasting colour to the container to which it is being applied

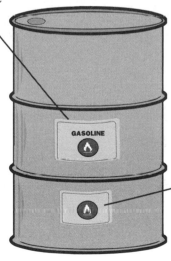

Workplace label— these are put on at the workplace. They include:

◆ product identifier

◆ safe handling procedures

◆ reference to MSDS being available

WHMIS class symbols

Class A–compressed gas

Class B–flammable and combustible materials

Class C–oxidizing materials

Class D—poisonous and infectious materials
division 1–materials having immediate and serious toxic effects

division 2–materials having other toxic effects

division 3–biohazardous infectious materials

Class E—corrosive material

Class F–dangerously reactive material

B

Safety at play

Canadians are active people, and sometimes it's when we're playing that we put ourselves at the greatest risk for injury. You can reduce your risk of injury by making these 5 smart choices

◆ buckle up—wear your seat belt. It greatly reduces your risk of being seriously hurt or killed in a collision. Buckle your climbing harness, your personal floatation device

◆ look first—whatever it is, look before you leap. When diving, mountain biking or jumping into the future, look first

◆ wear the gear—look at the gear the pros wear—they dress to protect themselves from injury so they can continue to compete. By wearing the correct gear for the activity you are engaged in, you'll reduce the chance of injuring yourself

◆ get trained—virtually everything we do at work and at play we can do better, and more safely, with training. Learn how to do it right by taking a lesson—this includes first aid training too

◆ drive sober—this means more than choosing to not drink and drive. It means 100% concentration on driving , with no distractions, whether you're driving a car, snowmobile or a motorbike

B

Just about everything we do involves some element of risk—risk ranging from what seems insignificant, like walking down a sidewalk, to risks none of us would take, like jumping in front of a moving train. In the middle, however, are risks that we can choose to take, or not take. Risk is personal and can vary day to day, depending on how tired you are, the weather conditions, even the time of day. Make your own choice on how much risk it makes sense for you to take at that moment.

Safety on the road

Take a defensive driving course

A defensive driving course is a good way to safety
check your driving. With professional training,
your chances of driving collision-free are much
improved. If you drive as part of your job, take a
refresher course for professional drivers every few years.
We can all use reminders to keep the bad habits away,
and it's a great way to learn of any changes to the rules of
the road.

Are you ready?

There are many conditions that will affect your next trip. If
you are driving, you will have to contend with variable
conditions of the road, light, weather, traffic, not to mention
the other drivers and vehicles. But the most important
condition is the condition of the driver—you! If you are
properly prepared to begin your journey (even a short one)
you will be able to compensate for other conditions that
are less than perfect.

Helping other motorists

If someone else is stopped
on the side of the road and
you think they need help,
pull over. Don't get out of
your car—open your window
just enough to talk.

Get information about the
problem and offer to go
and get help. Send police
or a service vehicle to the
scene.

Be prepared to drive before you get into the vehicle

Are you overtired or preoccupied? Is
your ability to react quickly impaired
by alcohol or drugs? What effect does
your prescription or over-the-counter
medication have on your abilities? Plan
your trip before your leave the
house and check expected weather
conditions. Review the plan with your
passengers so you won't have to consult
the map while driving.

B

Be sure your vehicle is well maintained

This includes both regular service and appropriate daily maintenance. Walk around your car before you get in it. Look for any signs of potential trouble. Are there lights that need replacing? Do the windshield wipers work properly and are all fluids topped up? Are there any fluids leaking underneath? Are all windows clean and completely clear of obstructions (ice, snow or mud)? Make sure all your lights are clear too.

Use seat belts and appropriate children's restraint systems (CRS)

Your seat belt gives you your best protection in a collision— wear it all the time. The lap belt must be worn low over your hips and adjusted so it feels snug. The shoulder belt should go over the shoulder and across the chest.

Infants and children must be properly fastened into a children's restraint system (CRS) fitted to their size and weight. Check the label on the CRS for the weight and height that are allowed. Infants should be in a rear-facing CRS appropriate for weight and height. A rear-facing infant-only restraint can safely restrain the infant up to a minimum 9-10 kg (20-22 lb). For heavier infants, use a rear-facing infant child restraint with a label that says it can be used for children who weigh more than 9-10 kgs in the rear-facing mode. The longer a child can stay rear-facing, the better. Forward-facing restraints need to be anchored by both the seat belt and the tether strap or by the Universal Anchorage System (UAS) and the tether strap. Check to make sure your CRS is properly anchored. Booster seats are used for children who weigh more than 18kgs (40 lbs). These seats are used to a minimum of 36 kg (80 lb). Always fasten your infant or

B

child into their CRS according to the directions that came with the CRS —if you don't, the CRS won't protect your child the way it's designed to. Never put a rear-facing infant seat into a front seat equipped with an airbag. Put the infant in the back seat.

Is your vehicle equipped for an emergency?

◆ an appropriate first aid kit
◆ booster cables
◆ flares or other warning devices
◆ candles with waterproof matches
◆ warm blankets
◆ extra clothing, including hats, mitts or gloves and warm boots
◆ high energy snacks

In case of a collision

◆ stay calm
◆ stay with your vehicle
◆ check yourself and anyone travelling with you—is anyone hurt?
◆ give first aid if required
◆ call police, if required
◆ exchange insurance information with other drivers involved
◆ before you leave the scene, be sure to write down the names, addresses and telephone numbers of any other drivers involved as well as witnesses to the collision

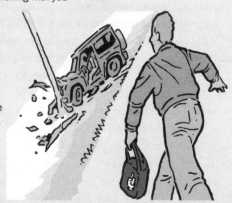

B

Be prepared

An emergency can happen any place, any time. With a little advance planning, you can be prepared for the unexpected. First, know what to do in an emergency—this means being trained in first aid. Second, make sure you have the materials you're going to need in an emergency—this means having first aid kits.

First aid training

As discussed on page 10, a good first aid course is the only way to learn the skills of first aid—and it is the skills that matter the most in an emergency. St. John Ambulance offers a wide variety of first aid courses—many of them are listed below. Why take a course from St. John Ambulance? St. John Ambulance first aid courses offer many advantages, including:

◆ highly trained instructors—St. John Ambulance instructors must be certified through our Instructor Development Program

◆ proven training techniques—our emergency and standard first aid courses, for example, are presented through a careful mix instructor-led activities, video demonstrations, instructor demonstrations and practice sessions

◆ flexible course content—many of our courses are based on the modular concept, so you can choose the topics most suited to your needs

◆ national certification—a St. John Ambulance first aid certificate is recognized across Canada

Selected St. John courses

First aid courses

◆ We can help—first aid training for kids

◆ The Lifesaver—a 3½-hour course for busy people

◆ Emergency First Aid—a 1-day course

◆ Standard First Aid—a 2-day course

◆ Medical First Responder

◆ Instructor Development Program

◆ Instructor-Trainer Development Program

◆ CPR courses

B

St. John Ambulance first aid kits

The reasons for owning a St. John Ambulance first aid kit are painfully obvious. Injuries can happen at home, at play or on the job. St. John Ambulance provides you with a full range of high-quality first aid kits for all types of injuries. Designed with you in mind our one-wound one-pack concept ensures quick and easy access to the tools you need in an emergency.

Family Kit—At home or at the cottage this kit contains the essential materials to deal with large, medium and small-sized wounds, as well as burns.

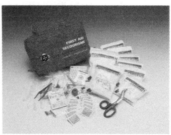

Vehicle Kit—Perfect for any vehicle this kit holds the necessary items to handle first aid on the road. Includes an SOS signal sign.

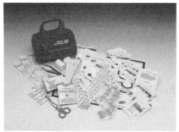

CPR Kit—Convenient key ring pouch design contains a disposable one-way valve CPR mask, wipes and gloves.

Sport Kit—From splints to cold compresses this kit contains the necessary first aid supplies to deal with sports injuries. Coaches and trainers will appreciate its compact size – easy to add to a gym or sport bag.

Compact Kit—Light and compact enough to be tucked into a backpack or looped onto a belt – perfect for the outdoors enthusiast. Contains the materials to tend to small and medium-sized wounds.

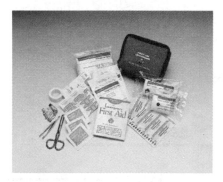

Fanny Kit—Essential outdoor gear for hiking, cycling, skiing and other activities. This weather-resistant fanny pack can be worn around the waist for easy access when dealing with small and medium-sized wounds.

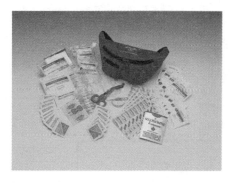

For more information or to purchase a kit contact your local St. John Ambulance office. Remember to restock your kit after you use it.

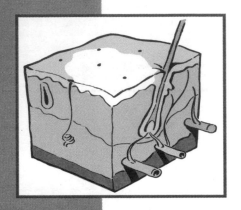

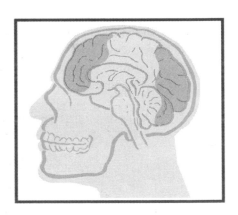

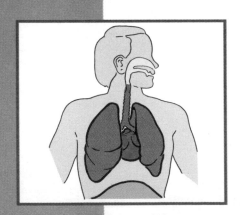

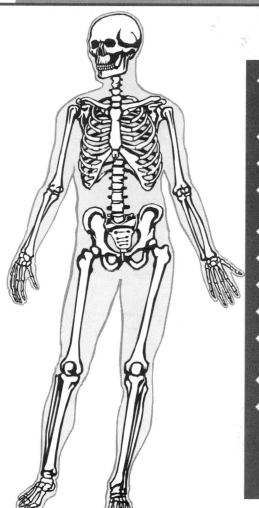

APPENDIX

C

THE BODY AND HOW IT WORKS

- ◆ *Introduction to anatomy and physiology*

- ◆ *Anatomical terms*

- ◆ *The skin*

- ◆ *Musculoskeletal system*

- ◆ *Joints*

- ◆ *Nervous system*

- ◆ *Brain*

- ◆ *Eyes*

- ◆ *Digestive and urinary systems*

- ◆ *Circulatory system*

- ◆ *Respiratory system*

Introduction to anatomy and physiology

As a first aider, you don't need a full knowledge of anatomy and physiology. However, you should know the basic structure of the human body and how it functions normally. This chapter describes the terms used in anatomy so that you can be more precise when giving information about a person's condition. It gives a short description of the major organs and functions of the skin, musculoskeletal system, nervous system including the eye, digestive and urinary, circulatory and respiratory systems.

Anatomical terms

These are the words used to describe where things are on the body and how they relate to each other.

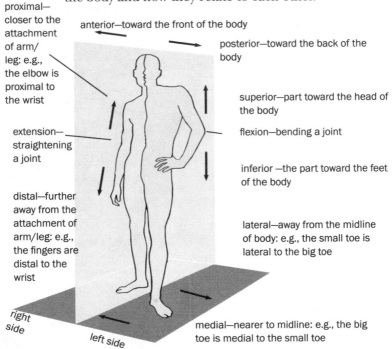

proximal—closer to the attachment of arm/leg: e.g., the elbow is proximal to the wrist

anterior—toward the front of the body

posterior—toward the back of the body

superior—part toward the head of the body

extension—straightening a joint

flexion—bending a joint

inferior —the part toward the feet of the body

distal—further away from the attachment of arm/leg: e.g., the fingers are distal to the wrist

lateral—away from the midline of body: e.g., the small toe is lateral to the big toe

right side

left side

medial—nearer to midline: e.g., the big toe is medial to the small toe

The skin

The skin is an important organ of the body. Its primary functions are to protect the body from environmental hazards and infection, eliminate waste in the form of sweat, help maintain normal body temperature and tell the brain of environmental temperature changes.

Environmental control

A rich supply of nerves in the skin keeps the brain aware of environmental changes. These nerves are sensitive to heat, cold, pain and touch, and they transmit these sensations to the brain. The skin helps the body adjust to its environment and protects it from extreme temperatures. In cold temperatures, blood vessels constrict to reduce blood flow near the surface of the skin. This helps prevent loss of heat from the body core. The fatty layers under the skin insulate the body to keep in body heat. In hot temperatures, the blood vessels near the skin surface dilate (get larger), allowing more blood flow near the skin. This cools the body by moving heat from the core to the surface, where it either radiates from the body, or is used to evaporate perspiration, having a cooling effect.

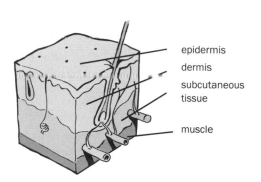

epidermis

dermis

subcutaneous tissue

muscle

Functions of the skin

◆ to protect the body from bacterial invasion

◆ to help control body temperature

◆ to retain body fluids

◆ to help eliminate waste products through perspiration

◆ to insulate the body

C

Musculoskeletal system

The musculoskeletal system is the framework of the body within which organs and body systems function. This framework includes bones, muscles, tendons and ligaments. Bones act as levers for muscle action; muscles shorten to produce movement; tendons attach muscles to bones; ligaments attach bones to bones at the joints. The musculoskeletal system protects organs, supports the body, and provides for its movement.

Muscles

Muscles are made of a special kind of tissue that contracts (shortens) when stimulated by nerve impulses. Generally, body movement is caused by several muscles working in combination—as some are contracting, others are relaxing. The nerves in the muscles carry impulses to and from the brain.

Muscles are classified as either voluntary or involuntary. Voluntary muscles are consciously controlled by the person, meaning they can be contracted or relaxed as the individual wishes. The muscles that move the skeleton are voluntary.

Involuntary muscles contract and relax rhythmically without any conscious effort on the part of the person. The heart, which has its own regulating system, is a good example of an involuntary muscle.

The diaphragm, a large dome-shaped muscle that separates the chest and abdominal cavities and is used in breathing, has characteristics of both voluntary and involuntary muscles. The contraction of this muscle, and thus the rate of breathing, can be changed at will for short periods of time.

diaphragm

Skeleton

The skeleton, made up of bones, forms the supporting structure that gives the body its shape. It also protects many of the organs—for example, the brain is protected by the skull, the heart and lungs by the ribs, and the spinal cord by the vertebrae.

The joints

The bones allow body movement by serving as rigid levers for tendons and muscles. The joints are formed where two or more bones come together. Immovable joints allow no movement, as in the

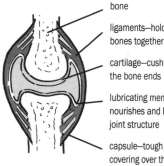

bone

ligaments—hold bones together

cartilage—cushions the bone ends

lubricating membrane—nourishes and lubricates the joint structure

capsule—tough covering over the joint

bones of the adult skull. Slightly movable joints allow only limited movement and are found between the vertebrae and between the pelvis and the spine. Freely moving joints are covered with smooth cartilage to minimize friction, and are held together by bands of strong tissue called ligaments.

Spine

The spine is divided into five parts as shown in the diagram. There are 33 bones in the spine, called vertebrae. The vertebrae stack on top of each other with discs between them. The discs are made of a tough flexible material and serve as shock absorbers in the spine. All the discs and vertebrae have an opening in the centre such that, when they stack together, there is a long channel that runs from the top to the bottom of the spine. The spinal cord, which carries all nerve impulses to and from the brain, runs through this channel. The spine protects the spinal cord, but if the spine is fractured, broken bones, displaced tissue and swelling can damage the spinal cord, possibly causing lifelong disability.

Parts of the spine

cervical
7 vertebrae

thoracic
12 vertebrae

lumbar
5 vertebrae

sacral
5 fused vertebrae

coccygeal
4 fused vertebrae
form the tailbone

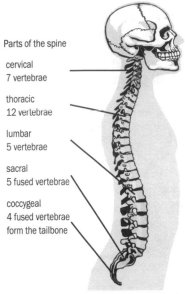

Thorax

The thorax is made up of the ribs, the 12 thoracic vertebrae and the sternum (breastbone). The thorax protects the organs in the chest, mainly the heart and lungs. It also provides some protection for the upper abdominal organs, including the liver at the front and the kidneys at the back. Injuries to the bones of the thorax threaten the organs they protect, and can therefore be life threatening.

ribs —12 pairs are attached to the vertebrae in back and either to the sternum, or to each other, in front. The lowest ribs attach to the vertebrae only, and are called "floating ribs"

sternum—a dagger-shaped bone with the point downward

xiphoid process (tip of sternum)—a strong piece of cartilage. Pressure on this cartilage can damage underlying organs

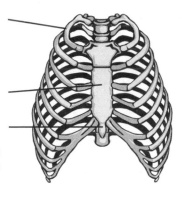

cranium—the plate-like bones fuse together during childhood to form a rigid case for the brain

facial bones join with bones of the cranium to form the eye and nose cavities which protect the eyes and nose

upper jaw (maxilla)

lower jaw (mandible)

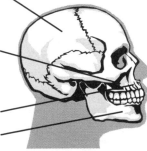

Skull

All the bones of the head make up the skull. The skull gives the head its shape and also protects the brain. When the skull is fractured, the brain may also be injured.

Main bones of the skeleton

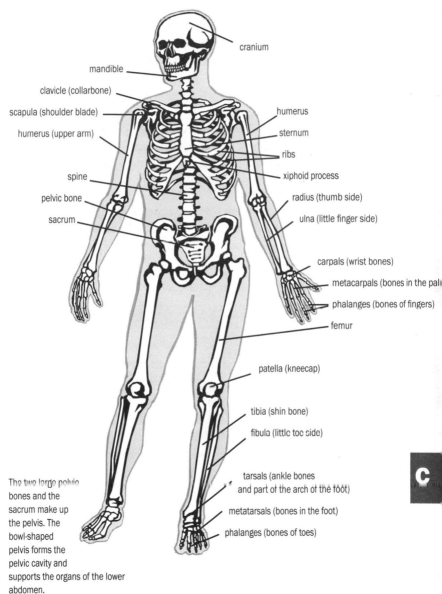

cranium

mandible

clavicle (collarbone)

scapula (shoulder blade)

humerus (upper arm)

humerus

sternum

spine

pelvic bone

sacrum

ribs

xiphoid process

radius (thumb side)

ulna (little finger side)

carpals (wrist bones)

metacarpals (bones in the pal

phalanges (bones of fingers)

femur

patella (kneecap)

tibia (shin bone)

fibula (little toe side)

tarsals (ankle bones
and part of the arch of the foot)

metatarsals (bones in the foot)

phalanges (bones of toes)

The two large pelvic bones and the sacrum make up the pelvis. The bowl-shaped pelvis forms the pelvic cavity and supports the organs of the lower abdomen.

C

Nervous System

The nervous system is composed of the brain, spinal cord and nerves. The brain and spinal cord together are called the central nervous system. The nerves that spread out to all parts of the body are called peripheral nerves. The nervous system is sub divided into the voluntary nervous system and the autonomic nervous system. The voluntary nervous system controls functions at the will of the individual. The autonomic nervous system controls functions without the conscious effort of the individual—e.g. heartbeat, breathing, blood pressure, digestion and glandular secretions such as hormones.

The peripheral nerves that extend from the spinal cord to all parts of the body are of two kinds—motor nerves and sensory nerves. Motor nerves control movement. Sensory nerves transmit sensations of touch, taste, heat, cold and pain to the brain.

Brain

The brain, the controlling organ of the body, occupies almost all the space in the cranium. It is the centre of consciousness, memory and thought. It receives information and transmits impulses to all parts of the body for voluntary and involuntary activities.

Eyes

The eye is the organ of sight. Any injury to the eye is potentially serious and may result in impaired vision or blindness. The quick response of the first aider and the correct first aid may help prevent permanent damage to the eye.

eyelid—movable layers of skin that provide a protective covering for the eye

iris—coloured set of muscles which control the size of the pupil, which in turn controls the amount of light entering the eye

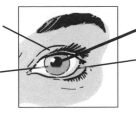

pupil—opening that lets light into the eye

conjunctiva—smooth, transparent membrane covering the front of the eye and Inner eyelids

cornea—thin, transparent front of the eyeball that allows light to enter the eye

aqueous humor—the watery fluid filling the space between the cornea and the iris

lens—changes shape to focus light rays upon the retina

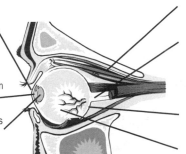

muscles—used to control eye movement

optic nerve—transmits nerve impulses to the brain for visual interpretation

retina—light-sensitive layer covering the back of the inside of the eye. It changes the light images into nerve impulses

vitreous humor —the clear, jelly-like fluid filling the cavity behind the lens

Digestive and urinary systems

The digestive and urinary systems convert food and drink into nutrients for the cells and collect and dispose of solid and fluid waste. The organs of these systems are classified as hollow or solid. The hollow, tubular organs carry digestive and urinary materials. The solid organs are tissue masses with a rich blood supply.

Injury to hollow organs may allow the contents to spill out into the abdominal or pelvic cavities, causing infection. Injury to the solid organs can result in severe internal bleeding.

C

Digestive system

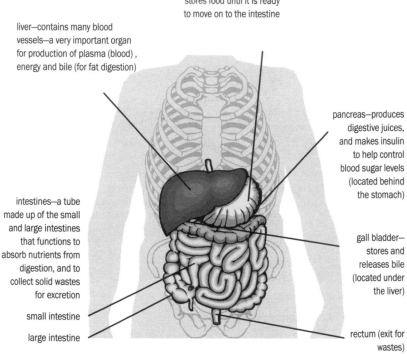

stomach—digests and stores food until it is ready to move on to the intestine

liver—contains many blood vessels—a very important organ for production of plasma (blood) , energy and bile (for fat digestion)

pancreas—produces digestive juices, and makes insulin to help control blood sugar levels (located behind the stomach)

intestines—a tube made up of the small and large intestines that functions to absorb nutrients from digestion, and to collect solid wastes for excretion

gall bladder— stores and releases bile (located under the liver)

small intestine

large intestine

rectum (exit for wastes)

C

Urinary system

The urinary system removes and collects waste products from the blood and eliminates them from the body in the form of urine. It is made up of the kidneys, ureters, bladder and urethra.

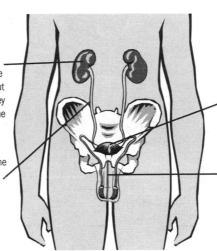

kidneys–huge quantities of blood pass through the kidneys which extract waste products and produce about 2500 mL of urine daily. They are partially protected by the lower ribs in the back

ureters–tubes that carries urine to the bladder from the kidneys

bladder–a sac which receives and holds urine until it is excreted

urethra–tube through which urine is excreted to the outside

Circulatory system

The circulatory system is a complex closed circuit consisting of the heart and blood that circulates blood throughout the body. Blood circulation is essential for distributing oxygen and nutrients to cells, and for collecting waste products from cells for excretion from the body.

Heart

The heart is a hollow, muscular organ about the size of a fist. It is located in the chest cavity behind the sternum. The heart functions as a two-sided pump, continuously pumping blood to the lungs and throughout the body. It pumps by first relaxing and filling up with blood, then contracting to squeeze or pump the blood out into the

C

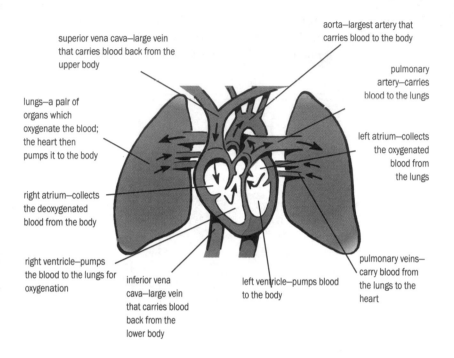

superior vena cava–large vein that carries blood back from the upper body

aorta–largest artery that carries blood to the body

pulmonary artery–carries blood to the lungs

lungs–a pair of organs which oxygenate the blood; the heart then pumps it to the body

left atrium–collects the oxygenated blood from the lungs

right atrium–collects the deoxygenated blood from the body

right ventricle–pumps the blood to the lungs for oxygenation

inferior vena cava–large vein that carries blood back from the lower body

left ventricle–pumps blood to the body

pulmonary veins–carry blood from the lungs to the heart

blood vessels. To make the heart beat effectively, it has a complex system of nerves. These nerves carry electrical impulses that control the beating of the heart.

Blood vessels

The blood travels through blood vessels. There are three main types of blood vessels: arteries, capillaries and veins. The arteries are the strongest blood vessels. They carry blood, under pressure, from the heart to all parts of the body. The arteries expand according to the volume of blood being forced through them by the pumping action of the heart, and return to normal size as the heart refills for the next contraction. This pressure wave can be felt as a pulse.

The largest artery, the aorta, emerges from the top of the heart. The coronary arteries branch off from the top of the aorta to supply the heart with blood. The smallest arteries are called arterioles and eventually form capillaries. Capillaries are the tiny blood vessels that reach every living cell to deliver oxygen, food, etc. and collect waste products. They have very thin walls to allow for the exchange of fluids and gases. Capillaries eventually join to form tiny venules, which in turn form veins. The veins take the blood back to the heart. Veins have thinner walls than arteries and most have cuplike valves that allow blood to flow only toward the heart.

Blood

Blood is the fluid that circulates through the heart and blood vessels. It transports oxygen and nutrients to the cells and carries away carbon dioxide and other waste products. Blood is composed of plasma, red cells, white cells and platelets—see sidebar.

Blood circulation

The blood circulation system is a closed loop beginning and ending at the heart. It consists of:

♦ pulmonary circulation—starting at the right side of the heart, blood is pumped to the lungs, where it drops off carbon dioxide and picks up oxygen, and then moves it back to the left side of the heart

♦ systemic circulation—starting at the left side of the heart, blood is pumped to the body, where it delivers oxygen and picks up carbon dioxide, and then moves it back to the right side of the heart

Blood components

♦ plasma—pale yellow liquid that carries cells, platelets, nutrients and hormones

♦ red blood cells—carry oxygen

♦ white blood cells—protect the body against microbes

♦ platelets—help form blood clots to stop bleeding

C

Blood pressure

Blood pressure is the pressure of the blood pushing against the inside walls of the blood vessels. With each heartbeat, there is a wave of pressure that travels throughout the circulatory system. The pressure wave is strong enough to be felt as a pulse at various points in the body, including the wrist (radial pulse), the neck (carotid pulse), and the upper arm (brachial pulse). Three factors control blood pressure:

◆ blood volume (how much blood is in the body)

◆ the capacity and elasticity of the blood vessels

◆ the strength of the heartbeat

If blood pressure is too low, the body's tissues don't get enough oxygen. This results in shock. Severe bleeding reduces the blood volume, which affects blood pressure. The body tries to compensate for blood loss by contracting the blood vessels and reducing the capacity of the circulatory system. With continued blood loss, however, the body cannot compensate and blood pressure drops. The casualty then starts showing signs of shock.

C

Respiratory system

The respiratory system causes air to be drawn into, and pushed out of, the lungs. The fresh air we breathe contains about 21% oxygen. In the lungs, blood picks up some of the oxygen and releases carbon dioxide. The air we breathe out has less oxygen (about 16%) and more carbon dioxide.

The respiratory system has three main parts: the airway, the lungs and the diaphragm. The airway is the passage which air follows to get from the nose and mouth to the lungs. In the lungs, blood drops off carbon dioxide and picks up oxygen. This process is called gas exchange. The diaphragm, a smooth, flat muscle just below the lungs, is used in breathing.

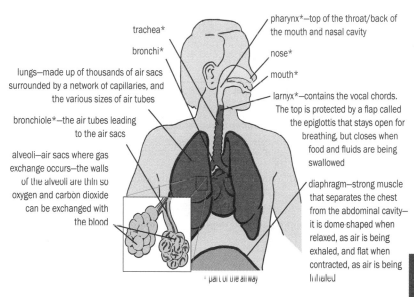

trachea*

bronchi*

lungs—made up of thousands of air sacs surrounded by a network of capillaries, and the various sizes of air tubes

bronchiole*—the air tubes leading to the air sacs

alveoli—air sacs where gas exchange occurs—the walls of the alveoli are thin so oxygen and carbon dioxide can be exchanged with the blood

pharynx*—top of the throat/back of the mouth and nasal cavity

nose*

mouth*

larnyx*—contains the vocal chords. The top is protected by a flap called the epiglottis that stays open for breathing, but closes when food and fluids are being swallowed

diaphragm—strong muscle that separates the chest from the abdominal cavity— it is dome-shaped when relaxed, as air is being exhaled, and flat when contracted, as air is being inhaled

* part of the airway

Respiratory control

Breathing is controlled by the respiratory centre in the brain, located near the base of the neck. It monitors the amount of oxygen and carbon dioxide in the blood. As the levels of oxygen and carbon dioxide change, the respiratory centre responds by changing the rate and depth of breathing.

How much oxygen is used, and how much carbon dioxide is given off, is related to the level of physical activity of the person. As physical activity goes up, more oxygen is used and more carbon dioxide is given off, so the respiratory centre increases the rate and depth of breathing to compensate (the heart rate also goes up). Breathing slows down when less oxygen is needed and less carbon dioxide is being produced.

Mechanism of breathing

The lungs have no way of drawing air into themselves. Instead, the diaphragm and the muscles between the ribs work together to expand the chest, which in turn expands the lungs. This causes air to be pulled into the lungs. As the breathing muscles relax, the chest returns to its smaller size and air is forced out of the lungs.

The lungs are covered with a smooth, slippery tissue called the pleural membrane. It is a continuous, double-layered tissue, one layer attached to the lungs and the other to the inside of the chest wall. The pleura acts as a lubricating layer to allow easy movement between the chest wall and the lungs, and to ensure that the lungs expand with the action of the chest wall.

C

Glossary

A

Abandonment: a first aider leaves the casualty without consent and without the care of a responsible person.

Abdominal thrust: the Heimlich manoeuvre; the manual thrusts to create pressure to expel an airway obstruction.

ABC's: Acronym meaning A= airway; B = breathing; C= circulation.

Abortion: the premature expulsion from the uterus of the products of conception.

Abrasion: a scraped or scratched skin wound.

Acute: a condition that comes on quickly, has severe symptoms and lasts a relatively short time.

Adam's apple: the bump on the front surface of the neck formed by part of the larynx (voice-box).

AED: Automated External Defibrillator- a device used to deliver a shock to help restart a stopped heart.

A.I.D.S.: *acquired immunodeficiency syndrome*; a fatal disease spread through the HIV (human immunodefiency virus).

Airway: the route for air in and out of the lungs.

Allergens: substances which trigger an allergic reaction in the body.

Allergic reaction: a hypersensitive response to normally harmless substances.

Alveoli: air sacs of the lungs.

Amniotic sac: a sac holding fluid surrounding a fetus in the uterus.

Amputation: complete removal of an appendage (leg, arm, finger, etc.).

Anaphylaxis: an exaggerated allergic reaction; may be rapidly fatal.

Anatomy: the structure of the body.

Angina (pectoris): a spasmodic pain in the chest due to a lack of blood supply to the heart.

Aorta: the largest artery in the body; originates at the left ventricle.

Aqueous humor: the watery fluid produced in the eye and located between the lens and the cornea.

Arteries: blood vessels that carry blood away from the heart.

Arteriosclerosis: a name for several conditions that cause the walls of the arteries to become thick, hard and inelastic.

ASA: acetylsalicylic acid—a medication available without prescription used to relieve pain, reduce swelling, reduce fever, etc.

Asthma: attacks of difficult breathing with wheezing/coughing, often due to allergens.

Atherosclerosis: a form of arteriosclerosis caused by fat deposits in the arterial walls.

Aura: a sensation of an impending seizure; may be a smell, taste, etc.

Autonomic nervous system: part of the nervous system that regulates involuntary functions (not controlled by conscious thought), such as pulse, breathing, digestion, hormone secretion, etc.

Avulsion: an injury where a piece of tissue is partially or completely torn away.

B

Back blows: sharp blows to the back, done to relieve an airway obstruction.

Bacteria: germs which can cause disease.

Bandage: material which holds a dressing in place

Basic life support (BLS): maintaining the ABC's without equipment (excluding barrier devices)

Blood clot: a semi-solid mass of blood products used by the body to stop bleeding.

Blood pressure: the pressure of blood against the walls of arterial blood vessels.

G

Blood volume: the total amount of blood in the heart and the blood vessels.

Bloody show: the mucous and bloody discharge signalling the beginning of labour.

Brachial pulse: pulse felt on the inner upper arm, normally taken on infants.

Breech birth: the delivery of a baby's buttocks or a foot first, instead of the head.

Bronchi: the main branches of the trachea carrying air into the lungs. Smaller branches called bronchioles.

Bronchospasm: severe tightening of the bronchi/bronchioles.

Bruise: broken blood vessels under the skin.

C

Capillaries: very small blood vessels that link the arteries and the veins; allow gases and nutrients to move into and out of the tissues.

Carbon dioxide (CO$_2$): a waste gas produced by the cells; an important stimulant for control of breathing.

Carbon monoxide (CO): a dangerous, colourless, odourless gas which displaces the carrying of oxygen by the red blood cells.

Cardiovascular disease: refers to disorders of the heart and blood vessels; e.g. high blood pressure and arteriosclerosis.

Cardiac arrest: the sudden stopping of cardiac function with no pulse, and unresponsiveness. In first aid, also means no breathing.

Carotid artery: the main artery of the neck; used to assess the carotid pulse.

Carpals: small bones of the wrist.

Cartilage: a tough, elastic tissue covering the surfaces where bones meet, also forms part of the nose, and ears.

Central nervous system: part of the nervous system consisting of the brain and the spinal cord.

Cerebrovascular accident (CVA): stroke; sudden stopping of circulation to a part of the brain.

Cervical collar: a device used to immobilize and support the neck.

Cervix: the lowest portion, or neck, of the uterus.

Chest thrusts: a series of manual thrusts to the chest to relieve an airway obstruction.

Cholesterol: a fatty substance found in animal tissue or products; also produced by the body; thought to contribute to arteriosclerosis.

Chronic: a condition with a long and/or frequent occurrence.

Chronic obstructive pulmonary disease (COPD): a term describing a group of lung diseases that cause obstructive problems in the airways: usually consists of chronic bronchitis, emphysema.

Circulatory system: the heart and blood vessels.

Clavicles: the collarbones.

Clonic phase: describes a convulsion where tightness and relaxation follow one another.

Closed wound: wound where the skin is intact.

Compression: is a condition of excess pressure on some part of the brain, usually caused by a buildup of fluids inside the skull.

Concussion: a temporary disturbance of brain function usually caused by a blow to the head or neck.

Congestive Heart Failure: failure of the heart to pump effectively, causing a back-up of fluid in the lungs and body tissues.

Conjunctiva: the transparent membrane covering the front of the eyeball (cornea) and the inner eyelids.

Contamination: contact with dirt, microbes, etc.

Contract: to shorten; usually refers to a muscle which exerts a pull when it shortens.

Convection: the loss of heat caused by the movement of air over the body.

COPD: Chronic obstructive pulmonary disease

(see above).

Cornea: the transparent front part of the eyeball.

Coronary artery: vessel which feeds the heart muscle.

Cranium: the part of the skull covering the brain.

Crepitus: the grating noise made when fractured bone ends rub together.

Croup: a group of viral infections that cause swelling of the inner throat.

Cyanosis: a bluish or gray colour of the skin due to insufficient oxygen in the blood.

D

Decapitation: the traumatic removal of the head.

Defibrillation: applying an electrical shock to a fibrillating heart.

Deoxygenated blood: blood containing a low level of oxygen.

Dermis: the inner layer of the skin containing hair germinating cells, sweat glands, nerves and blood vessels.

Diabetes: a disease caused by insufficient insulin in the blood; causes excessive blood sugar.

Diaphragm: a large dome-shaped muscle separating the chest and abdominal cavities.

Diarrhea: excessive watery bowel movements.

Direct pressure: force applied directly on a wound to help stop bleeding.

Dislocation: when the bone surfaces at a joint are no longer in proper contact.

Distal: refers to a part that is farther away from the attachment of a leg/arm/finger/toe.

Dressing: a covering over a wound, used to stop bleeding and prevent contamination of the wound.

E

Embedded object: an object stuck onto the surface (usually on the eye) or impaled into tissues.

Embolus: any foreign matter such as a blood clot, fat clump or air bubble carried in the blood stream.

Emetic: a substance used to cause vomiting.

E.M.S.: Emergency Medical Services system—a community's group of services which respond to emergencies including police, fire fighters, paramedics.

Emphysema: a chronic lung disease characterized by overstretched alveolar walls. See COPD.

Epidermis: The outermost layer of the skin.

Epiglottis: a lid-like piece of tissue which protects the entrance to the larynx (voice-box).

Epiglottitis: an infection usually in children resulting in a swelling of the epiglottis —may cause an airway obstruction.

Epilepsy: a chronic brain disorder characterized by recurrent convulsions.

E.S.M.: Emergency Scene Management—the sequence of actions a first aider should follow to give safe and appropriate first aid.

Exhalation: expiration; breathing out.

Extrication: freeing from being trapped (usually a car collision).

F

Femur: the thigh bone.

Fibrillation: uncoordinated contractions of the heart muscle, so that the blood out-flow is almost nil.

Fibula: the bone of the lower leg on the little toe side.

Flail chest: a condition in which several ribs are broken in at least two places, allowing a free-floating segment.

Flexion: bending a joint.

G

First aid: the help given to an injured or suddenly ill person using readily available materials.

First aider: someone who takes charge of an emergency scene and gives first aid.

Fracture: a broken or cracked bone

Frostbite: tissue damage due to exposure to cold.

G

Gallbladder: a sac under the liver that concentrates and stores bile; used for fat digestion.

Gastric distention: a swelling of the stomach usually with air, due to ventilating with excessive volume or force during artifical respiration.

Gauze: an open mesh material used for dressings.

Glasgow Coma Scale (modified): a method of estimating the casualty's level of consciousness.

Guarding: a tightening of the abdominal muscles when the casualty has abdominal pain and is touched there.

H

Head-tilt chin-lift manoeuvre: opening the casualty's airway by tilting the head backward and lifting the chin forward.

Heart attack: chest pain due to a death of a part of the heart muscle; a myocardial infarction.

Heart failure: a weakened heart muscle that is unable to push blood forward; it backs up into the lungs and also causes swelling of the ankles, etc.

Heat cramps: painful muscle spasms due to excessive loss of fluid and salts by sweating.

Heat exhaustion: excessive sweating causing a loss of water and salts.

Heat stroke: A life-threatening emergency where the temperature regulation mechanism cannot cool the body, and the temperature is far above normal—also called hyperthermia or sunstroke

Heimlich manoeuvre: abdominal thrusts done to remove an airway obstruction.

History: information about the casualty's problem: symptoms, events leading up to the problem, applicable illnesses or medications, etc.

Hyperglycemia: abnormally elevated blood sugar.

Hypertension: high blood pressure.

Hyperthermia: too high body temperature.

Hyperventilation: too deep and rapid respirations.

Hypoglycemia: too low blood sugar levels.

Hypothermia: too low body temperature.

Hypoxia: too low levels of oxygen in the body tissues.

I

Impaled object: an object which remains embedded in a wound.

Immobilization: placing some type of restraint along a body part to prevent movement.

Incontinence: loss of bladder and bowel control.

Infarction: an area of tissue death due to lack of blood flow.

Infection: inflammation due to microbes.

Inflammation: a tissue reaction to irritation, illness or injury; shows as redness, heat, swelling, and pain.

Inhalation: breathing in; inspiration.

Insulin: hormone produced by the pancreas; important in the regulation of blood sugar levels.

Insulin coma/reaction/shock: hypoglycemia (too low blood sugar levels) due to excessive insulin.

Intrapleural space: a tiny space containing a negative pressure (vacuum) between the two pleural layers.

Involuntary muscle: muscles not under conscious control; heart, intestines etc.

Iris: coloured part of the eye; made of muscles which control light entering the eye.

Ischemic: lacking sufficient oxygen; as in ischemic heart disease.

J

Joint: a place where two or more bones meet.

Joint capsule: a tough covering over a joint.

K

Kidneys: a pair of organs which filter blood and produce urine.

L

Labour: the muscular contractions of the uterus which expel the fetus.

Laceration: a jagged wound from a rip or a tear.

Laryngectomy: removal of the larynx (voice-box); results in a neck-breather.

Lens: a part of the eye which focuses light rays on the retina.

Ligament: a tough cord of tissue which connects bone to bone.

Lipoproteins: substances floating in the blood; made of proteins and fats.

Lymph: a fluid similar to plasma that circulates in the lymphatic system.

Lymphatic system: a system of vessels, nodes and organs which collects strayed proteins leaked from blood vessels and cleanses the body of microbes and other foreign matter.

M

Mandible: the bone of the lower jaw.

Mechanism of injury: the force that causes an injury and the way it is applied to the body.

Medical alert: a means of identifying casualties (usually a bracelet, necklace) who have a condition that may alter first aid treatment.

Medical help: the treatment given by or under the supervision of a medical doctor, e.g. ambulance attendant.

Metacarpals: bones of the palm of the hand.

Metatarsals: bones of the arch of the foot; between the ankle and toes.

Micro-organisms: germs which can cause illness.

Miscarriage: the lay term for an abortion; the loss of the products of conception.

Mouth-to-mouth ventilation: artificial respiration by blowing air into the mouth of the casualty .

Mucous membrane: thin, slick, transparent lining, covering tubes and cavities that open to the outside; the inner surface of the mouth, nose, eye, ear, rectum, etc.

Musculoskeletal system: all of the bones, muscles, and connecting tissues which allow locomotion (movement of the body).

Myocardial infarction: death of part of the cardiac (heart) muscle; heart attack.

N

Nail bed test: a method of assessing the adequacy of circulation to the extremities; gentle pressure is exerted on the nail bed until the tissue whitens; the return of colour to the area is assessed upon pressure release.

Negligence: failure to perform first aid at the level expected of someone with similar training and experience.

Nerve: a cord made up of fibres which carry nerve impulses to and from the brain.

Nervous system: the brain, spinal cord and nerves which control the body's activities.

Nitroglycerin: a drug used to ease the workload on the heart; often carried as a pill or spray by casualties with angina.

O

O$_2$: the chemical symbol for oxygen.

Obstructed airway: a blockage in the air passageway to the lungs.

Oxygen: an odourless, colourless gas essential to life.

P

Pancreas: an organ located under the stomach; produces digestive enzymes and hormones which regulate blood sugar.

Paralysis: inability to move a part; loss of motor function.

Patella: the bone of the knee cap.

Phalanges: bones of the fingers and toes.

Pharynx: the back of the mouth and above the voice box (larynx); a passageway for both air and food.

Physiology: the study of functions of the body.

Placenta: an organ attached to the uterus which provides a fetus with nourishment.

Plasma: a pale yellow fluid containing blood cells, nutrients, gases and hormones.

Platelet: a small, cell-like blood element important in blood clotting.

Pleural membrane: a slick membrane covering the outside surface of the lungs and the inside surface of the chest cavity (thorax).

Pneumonia: inflammation of the lungs.

Pneumothorax: an accumulation of air in the pleural space. Normally the pleural space contains a negative pressure or a vacuum; the air mass (instead of a vacuum) collapes the lung under it.

Position of function: refers to the position an injured hand is placed in when bandaged and/or splinted; i.e. fingers are gently curved with palm slightly downwards.

Primary survey: a step of ESM—assessing the casualty for life-threatening injuries and giving appropriate first aid.

Proximal: refers to a part that is closest to the attachment of a leg/arm/finger/toe/intestine.

Pulmonary artery: the major artery emerging from the right ventricle; carries deoxygenated blood to the lungs.

Pulse: the rhythmic expansion and relaxation of the arteries caused by the contractile force of the heart; usually felt where the vessels cross a bone near the surface.

R

Radiate: the spreading of something; the pain of a heart attack in the chest radiates to the left arm.

Radius: the bone on the thumb side of the lower arm.

Red blood cells: the most numerous type of blood cells; carry oxygen.

Respiratory arrest: stopped breathing.

Retina: the covering at the back of the eyeball; changes light rays into nerve impulses.

Reye's Syndrome: A rare but serious disease in children and adolescents that is reported to be associated with taking ASA for a viral infection. Reye's Syndrome affects the brain, liver and blood. It can cause permanent brain damage or death.

R.I.C.E.: R=rest; I= Immobilize; C= Cold; E= elevation. First aid for certain bone and joint injuries.

Rule of Nines: a system of estimating the amount of skin surface burned.

S

Sacrum: a bone formed from five fused vertebra; forms the back of the pelvis.

Scapula: shoulder blade.

Scene survey: the initial step of ESM (emergency scene management) where the first aider takes control, assesses any hazards and makes the area safe, finds out what has happened, identifies self as a first aider, gains consent from the casualty, calls for help from bystanders and starts organizing them to get help for the casualty.

Sclera: the white of the eye; the tough, opaque layer of the eyeball.

Secondary survey: a step of ESM; assessing the casualty for non-life-threatening injuries and giving appropriate first aid.

S.I.D.S. (Sudden Infant Death Syndrome): death of an infant due to unexplainable causes.

Sign: objective evidence of disease or injury.

Sling: a support for an arm or shoulder, usually brought around the neck.

Spleen: an organ of the lymphatic system; functions to cleanse foreign matter from the blood; blood reservoir.

Spontanoeus pneumothorax: air in the pleural space due to an unexplained rupture of the underlying lung.

Splint: is a rigid and padded support used to prevent movement in a bone or joint injury.

Sprain: supporting tissues about a joint (such as ligaments) are stretched, partly or completely torn.

Sternum: the breastbone.

Stoma: an opening in the neck through which the person breathes.

Strain: a stretched or torn muscle.

Sucking chest wound: a wound in which air is pulled into the chest cavity through the chest wall; it can cause a collapse of the lung beneath.

Superficial: on the surface of the body; as opposed to deep.

Superior vena cava: one of the two largest veins; it drains the arms and head of deoxygenated blood and empties into the right atrium.

Symptom: an indication of illness or injury experienced by a casualty; cannot be detected by an observer without asking.

Syrup of ipecac: an emetic; used to cause vomiting.

T

Tendon: a tough cord of tissue that attaches muscles to bones or other tissues.

Tension pneumothorax: air in the pleural space presses on the heart and blood vessels and affects their function.

Tetanus: a type of bacteria in a wound; can cause severe muscle spasms.

TIA: Transient ischemic attack: a mini-stroke.

Tibia: the bone in the lower leg; on the large toe side; the shin bone.

Tonic phase: first stage of a convulsion where the muscles are rigid.

Tourniquet: a constricting band used to stop severe bleeding.

Trachea: a tube for air, kept open with cartilage rings; is located between the larynx (voice-box) and the bronchi.

Traction: gently but firmly pulling below a fracture to bring the limb into alignment.

Transient ischemic attack (TIA): temporary signs and symptoms of a stroke due to a lack of sufficient oxygen to the brain.

Trauma: any physical or psychological injury.

Triage: a system of placing priorities for first aid and/or transportation for multiple casualties.

U

Ulna: bone in the lower arm; on the little finger side.

Urethra: a tube which carries urine from the bladder to the outside.

Uterus: the muscular sac which holds, protects a fetus.

V

Vein: a blood vessel; carries blood to the heart.

Ventilation: supplying air to the lungs.

Ventricles: the muscular lower chambers of the heart which pump blood into the arteries.

Ventricular fibrillation: a quivering action of the heart muscles so that little blood is pumped.

G

Vital signs: the four signs that show the basic condition of the casualty: level of consciousness; breathing; pulse; skin condition and temperature (sources vary as to the components of vital signs).

W

White blood cells: blood cells which are involved in immunity and control of microbes.

X

Xiphoid process: the cartilage tip at the lower end of the breastbone.

G

Index

A

B

I